FILM

ARTS FOR HEALTH

Series Editor: Paul Crawford, Professor of Health Humanities, University of Nottingham, UK

The *Arts for Health* series offers a ground-breaking set of books that guide the general public, carers and healthcare providers on how different arts can help people to stay healthy or improve their health and wellbeing.

Bringing together new information and resources underpinning the health humanities (that link health and social care disciplines with the arts and humanities), the books demonstrate the ways in which the arts offer people worldwide a kind of shadow health service – a non-clinical way to maintain or improve our health and wellbeing. The books are aimed at general readers along with interested arts practitioners seeking to explore the health benefits of their work, health and social care providers and clinicians wishing to learn about the application of the arts for health, educators in arts, health and social care and organizations, carers, and individuals engaged in public health or generating healthier environments. These easy-to-read, engaging short books help readers to understand the evidence about the value of arts for health and offer guidelines, case studies, and resources to make use of these non-clinical routes to a better life.

Other titles in the series:

Reading	Philip Davis and Fiona Magee
Theatre	Sydney Cheek-O'Donnell
Singing	Yoon Irons and Grenville Hancox
Music	Eugene Beresin
Painting	Victoria Tischler
Dancing	Sara Houston
Drawing	Curie Scott
Storytelling	Michael Wilson

FILM

DR STEVEN SCHLOZMAN

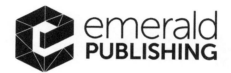

United Kingdom – North America – Japan – India
Malaysia – China

Emerald Publishing Limited
Howard House, Wagon Lane, Bingley BD16 1WA, UK

First edition 2021

Reprints and permissions service
Contact: permissions@emeraldinsight.com

British Library Cataloguing in Publication Data
A catalogue record for this book is available from the British Library

ISBN: 978-1-83867-312-3 (Print)
ISBN: 978-1-83867-309-3 (Online)
ISBN: 978-1-83867-311-6 (Epub)

INVESTOR IN PEOPLE

DEDICATION

This book is dedicated to George A. Romero for showing me that there is no better medicine than movies and a laugh.

CONTENTS

SERIES PREFACE: CREATIVE PUBLIC HEALTH

The "Arts for Health" series aims to provide key information on how different arts and humanities practices can support, or even transform, health, and wellbeing. Each book introduces a particular creative activity or resource and outlines its place and value in society, the evidence for its use in advancing health and wellbeing, and cases of how this works. In addition, each book provides useful links and suggestions to readers for following-up on these quick reads. We can think of this series as a kind of shadow health service – encouraging the use of the arts and humanities alongside all the other resources on offer to keep us fit and well.

Creative practices in the arts and humanities offer a fantastic, non-medical, but medically relevant way to improve the health and wellbeing of individuals, families, and communities. Intuitively, we know just how important creative activities are in maintaining or recovering our best possible lives. For example, imagine that we woke up tomorrow to find that all music, books, or films had to be destroyed, learn that singing, dancing, or theatre had been outlawed or that galleries, museums, and theaters had to close permanently; or, indeed, that every street had posters warning citizens of severe punishment for taking photographs, drawing, or writing. How would we feel? What would happen to our bodies and minds? How would we survive? Unfortunately, we have seen this kind of removal of creative activities from human society before and today many people remain terribly restricted in artistic expression and consumption.

I hope that this series adds a practical resource to the public. I hope people buy these little books as gifts for family and friends, or for hard-pressed healthcare professionals, to encourage them to revisit or to consider a creative path to living well. I hope that creative public health makes for a brighter future.

Professor Paul Crawford

ACKNOWLEDGMENTS

Countless conversations, endless e-mails, single line quips from film and TV ... this is the fodder from which I drew inspiration. But who created this fodder? My friends and family, of course. So, thank you, Ruta, Sofia, and Naomi. You've indulged me on both big and small screens alike. Thank you, Heather, for calling me with quotations every time you rewatch the Princess Bride. Thanks Mom and Dad, for letting the Wicked Witch of the West scare the pants off of me. And thanks Eric and Christina, for allowing me to wax almost poetic about campy stories. To Paul Crawford, who has tirelessly championed a good tale as the best kind of healing. To Larry Fessenden, for showing me that meaning is everywhere. To Adam Hart, for showing me that you can be scholarly about 1980s slasher films. To my buddy Peter, who introduced me to Jonah on SHH and who adores Terrence Malick. And to the students I've taught – for allowing me to see film through all of your eyes. Finally, to all of those who told their stories. May you never stop.

INTRODUCTION – WHY FILM?

Life is complicated.

This might seem a rather trite way to begin a book with the otherwise grand aspirations to summarize the relationship of film to health. However, think of this sentiment as a universal truth that is so terribly obvious that we sometimes fail to fully consider the richness of all that it implies. After all, we behave in maddeningly unpredictable ways.

We feel better when we feel sad. We frequently eat too much. We have been known to misbehave. We succeed without trying and we try often with no reasonable chance of success. The most perplexing fact of all is that we represent our peculiarities through the metaphors that art affords. *Why would we want to relive our oddness any more than we do in real life?* What could possibly be the reasons to explain our uniquely human tendency to represent ourselves, over and over, in artistic expression? Haven't we had enough?

Before we even get into the meat of this book's discussion, let us at least be clear about the following statement: *We need art.* This book fully agrees with the stringently held set of beliefs that we require art to tolerate the ebbs and flows of our very existence. Once we accept this premise, then we must further acknowledge that among the most fundamental of these ebbs and flows are the rocky waters of sickness and health. These forces hold enormous sway over all that we do and indeed all that we are. Art, we argue, is uniquely suited to capture and to convey the nuanced emotional experiences that characterize our daily struggles toward remaining healthy and whole.

1

This book, however, cannot capture all forms of art. To summarize the role of art in our quest for health is in fact the goal of the entire volume of books to which this small contribution belongs. Nevertheless, it is the premise of this volume that a case can be made that film is the most effective form of artistic expression for these lofty endeavors. In fact, one can argue that film, whether it appears in our theaters or our living rooms, is the most influential form of art throughout the world. Film, after all, remains popular in the developed and the developing world. Movies and television programs are discussed in the ivory towers of academia and across the bedlam of social media. One can literally read a discussion of the same film in a high brow journal and on the stalls of a public restroom. Debates about film are universally digested. No other form of artistic expression so completely dominates our cultural landscape. In this sense, film is the most available and accessible form of artistic expression. Indeed, the very breadth of film's reach makes the creation of this book somewhat daunting. How does one capture all that film offers in the service of staying well? I will without question fail to touch on every salient point. That is the risk of this kind of endeavor. There will be movies unmentioned and themes unexplored. I beg the reader's forgiveness now for these inevitable mishaps, and it is my great hope that readers will continue the discussions that have their genesis in the pages that follow.

Let's think for a moment about the ways that we allow film to permeate our daily existence. At the forefront of this discussion is the unusually intimate relationship we enjoy with the artists who create our on-screen stories. After all, how often can you recall or even access an interview with a famous artist whose work you enjoyed at a local gallery? How many speeches have you appreciated from the author of a favorite novel? In what form of art other than film can one see the artists themselves so willingly explain their thinking? These inquiries require only a rudimentary Internet search. Screenwriters, directors, cinematographers, actors, and producers are willing to share with all of us their experiences in the creation of the stories that unfold on the silver screens in our theaters and across the streaming networks in our homes. To this end, film enjoys enormous and unchallenged power to influence how we feel about ourselves and about each other.

Film can express for us the feelings that we have when we fall in love, when we are full of rage, when we marvel at the growth of our children, and when we slow down and eventually expire. We experience the trials and tribulations of the characters in every story that we see unfolding on screen. We are sometimes even moved to action by the activism of the stories themselves. Virtually every developed nation has its own set of awards to recognize excellence in the creation of movies and television, and the award ceremonies at these gala events inevitably discuss the gifts of understanding that on-screen stories afford. In short, film allows us to illustrate and therefore to celebrate the endlessly fascinating features of what it means to be human.

All of this is possible because films tell uniquely immersive stories. Neuroscientists and cultural commenters have described film as a kind of hypnosis; we find ourselves, without realizing it, experiencing the feelings of another person. In short, we become the characters on the screen. Somebody flinches in pain, and we in the audience flinch ourselves. When a character cries, we find ourselves crying. The ancient Greeks understood this well and called the strange transference of feelings from story to recipient as cathartic, a term that literally connotes a kind of cleansing. I argue that no other modality allows this cleansing as completely as film. This is true for fictional narratives and it is true for historical re-creations. This is true even for documentaries. In all of these forms of expression, we find ourselves emotionally invested. As a result, we are invited to better explore our own fears and our own celebrations. What better tool for the exploration of the human condition itself?

But why does all of this happen? Should we accept at face value that the experiences that film engenders necessarily allow us to better understand ourselves? How do we know that we do not simply leave the theater, or turn off our computers, or perhaps push the off button on the coffee table remote, and then simply go back to being who we were before we immersed ourselves in the experience?

The easy answer is that we should *not* accept this as a central and immutable tenet. It is entirely possible that many of us find ourselves unmoved by all that we see in the screen. However, current scientific inquiries find that this conclusion is increasingly unlikely. Our brains are rewarded handsomely when we allow ourselves to pursue our need to connect with one another. We are pack animals. We need to understand, therefore, the motivations of our pack. This understanding stems from a special interplay between sympathy and empathy. We will discuss these concepts as they relate to film later in this book. However, before we delve into the science, it makes sense to establish the unique method through which films manage to make us care so deeply.

I would like to argue that there exists a process through which we take in our movies and television programs. We start with the experience of sympathy. We *feel* for the "other," and in this case is the "other" is a character that we watch on the screen. This allows us to begin to close the chasm between the "other" and the "self." Because of this response, we desire to help or to assist or even to stop the characters to whom we are introduced from whatever we see unfolding in the narrative we are experiencing. Even more importantly, these desires take us deeper into our personal experiences, and because of these more intimate feelings, we move through an exploration of our sympathies into more intense experiences that promote empathic connectedness. Not only do we feel for the other, but we move toward feeling what the other feels. *We walk in the shoes of the other*. We go from feeling for a character to feeling as if we *are* that character.

These experiences ultimately lead to the wonders offered by the act of displacement. *For the purposes of this book, displacement is essentially a defense mechanism*. It is a tool that allows for the safe exploration of aspects of ourselves that we might otherwise feel uncomfortable experiencing more directly. We can understand our rage when we watch The Sopranos. We can understand love when we watch A Room with a View. We start by feeling for the "other" and then as we become more immersed we become the "other." As a result, we learn more about our own unique characteristics that were perhaps previously unknown, unrealized, or unappreciated. This is the magnificent sleight-of-hand that film affords.

Ultimately, through imagination, through the creation of sympathy, and through the engenderment of empathy, film fosters escapism. We leave our bodies through the experience of film and movies. Because of its immersive and hypnotic nature, film is among the most reliable and common forms of escape. To the extent that this kind of escapism has been shown to have strong associations with decreased stress, improvement in emotional health, and the preservation of psychological well-being, we can argue that for many people, film can function as a central aspect of emotional balance.

It follows, therefore, that film helps us with our physical health as well as our mental health. After all, mind and body are the same. The brain is connected to the rest of the body. A healthy mind is necessary for a healthy body, just as a healthy body makes possible the appreciation for emotional and psychological well-being. In some instances, it is possible that the positive effects of film work faster than almost any traditional therapeutic endeavors. There are studies documenting the extent to which people feel immediately better after enjoying a well told story on-screen. There is even research documenting the correlation between the appreciation of a good movie and an increased ability to fight infection. Importantly, these stories need not be uplifting. They must only be transformative and authentic. Because humans are themselves complex creatures, there will inevitably exist certain films that are more helpful for certain people. There is, one can argue, an on-screen story for everyone. By the same token, however, precisely because of our willingness to allow the immersion that film encourages, on-screen stories can also be traumatic and physically harmful. There are movies known for provoking nightmares and actual illnesses. Those same films are for others inspiring and health-inducing. Such is the complexity of diversity when it comes to our unique relationship to art of all forms.

Finally, there is a growing literature on the use of film to tolerate the discomfort of healthcare itself. Movies are shown during procedural medicine, such as dental work, to help children to tolerate chronic pain. The hypnotic nature of stories on-screen can distract us from the suffering that characterizes our endeavors to become healthier, and can help us to understand the sickness and suffering of others.

All of this is to say that film is core to our well-being. If we imagine a world where artistic expressions on screen were to suddenly disappear, it is my contention that this world would be characterized by significantly worse overall health. Film helps us to feel whole.

Because I am a physician, I tend to think of challenges in terms of sickness and health. Throughout the pages that follow, therefore, we will systematically make the case for film in the service of health, and we will discuss as well the ways that film can in some instances be harmful. We will start with the conditions which films help us to better understand. These include mental and physical illnesses as well as the ups and downs of everyday life. We will then move to discuss the ways that film helps to demonstrate and inspire the maintenance of wellness and the cohesion of otherwise diverse communities. These points will be illustrated through vignettes created from combinations of patient-care experiences that I have encountered personally or that have been relayed to me throughout my professional career. Importantly, these cases will span the life cycle. If we are to argue that film has the capacity to reach all ages, then our examples must draw from every stage of human development. Finally, we will end with recommendations for people in need and for those who care for them. Because we humans often hold both of these roles at various points in our lives, the recommendations put forth are transitive. Those who care for others and those are in turn cared for can easily change places, and the utility of film ought to speak to each of the important roles.

However, we must remember that there are challenges in the use of film as a tool to promote health. There are obstacles to overcome and barriers to cross. More research is needed to make full use of the utility of film. The final section of this book will discuss next steps toward a better understanding of the power of film as force for health.

1

DEPICTIONS OF ILLNESS IN MODERN CINEMA AND TELEVISION

As I have already noted, because I am a physician, it makes the most sense for me to construct this book through a somewhat medical lens. We will therefore begin by discussing the myriad ways that specific illnesses are depicted on screen. A unifying feature of virtually all scholarship exploring the relationship of art to healing is the extent to which artistic depictions of suffering can foster understanding of illness and health.

We are hard pressed, for example, to offer a cohesive and encompassing definition of illness, but we have much less room for disagreement when we witness illnesses in the context of a compelling on-screen narrative. Depictions of sickness in movies and television can foster understanding, sympathy, and empathy. Moreover, it appears that the willingness to include stories of sickness has increased in the film canon over the last few decades.

This is especially the case for emotional suffering. Past representations of these issues have long been relegated to largely stigmatizing depictions. We have seen through much of modern cinema our share of psychotic murderers, personality disordered relationship-wreckers, substance abusing sociopaths, and anxiety ridden anti-heroes. However, there is evidence that the tide is slowly shifting. Increasingly we are seeing carefully nuanced films that still manage to convey the dramatic appeal that psychological conditions bring to a story but that also introduce more authentic layers of complexity that allow us to better understand and experience empathy for the characters to whom we are introduced. The 2015 film *Silver Lining Playbook* is a perfect example of this new breed of film. Consider the fact that this remarkable movie manages to convey the challenges of bipolar disorder in Bradley Cooper's character and perhaps borderline personality disorder in Jennifer Lawrence's character while at the same time creating a bond between the audience and the characters. This is a far cry from the fairly one-sided and terrifying depictions in past films such as the portrayal of borderline personality disorder in *Fatal Attraction* or the homicidal rage in wonderful but for our purposes highly flawed stories such as *Psycho* or *Cape Fear*.

Throughout this chapter, we will discuss films that have been instrumental in helping us to better understand psychological suffering and especially specific psychiatric disorders, and then we will move to a discussion of non-psychiatric illnesses. I will also offer examples of the ways that films have served as potent therapeutic tools. Importantly, we will not limit our survey to recent films or to the relatively narrow focus of simply outlining the criteria for specific conditions and then applying these criteria to the characters in the movies we discuss. Instead, where possible we will examine movies that feature characters who are both medically diagnosable and at the same time lend themselves to thematic interpretations for their struggles.

Given the fact that literally thousands of pages have been written about the depiction of emotional challenges in film and television, our discussions will focus on the merits of only a few films. These particular films uniquely impact our understanding of and empathy for conditions such as depression and bipolar disorder. In later chapters, we will discuss filmic depictions of autism, anxiety, psychosis, and substance abuse. For this chapter, I have chosen unipolar depression and bipolar disorder because they are among the most common psychiatric disorders in the general population. We will then move to an examination of on-screen narratives that focus on non-psychiatric illnesses. It is my hope that these films will inspire readers to look for similar thematic trends in the increasing breadth of on-screen entertainment that our modern world offers. To this end, at the conclusion of this chapter, I will offer suggestions for additional films that address a host of different conditions.

MOOD DISORDERS AND FILM

Mood disorders constitute a wide range of psychiatric diagnoses. These include clinical depression, sometimes called unipolar depression, and the much less common condition of bipolar disorder, also called manic depressive illnesses. When examining on-screen depictions of mood disorders, it is a curious but understandable observation that there are more films about bipolar disorder even though the rate of unipolar depression in the general population is estimated to be at least 15 times more common than manic depressive illness. Perhaps this is best explained by the symptoms themselves. Whereas unipolar depression is more often characterized by low energy, decreased emotional expression, increased sleep and potential suicidality, mania, the core feature of bipolar disorder, features dramatic flourishes such as grandiose ideas, promiscuity and impulsive behavior that some would argue are better suited for on-screen storytelling. To some extent, the over-representation of bipolar disorder in films and television programs might lead some to believe that depression is much less common than mania. This is an example of the ways that art of all kinds, but especially widely consumed art, can affect public perceptions.

Consider the 2007 film *Michael Clayton*. The movie is universally celebrated as a riveting legal thriller that hinges on the titular protagonist, played by George Clooney, convincing his clearly manic law partner portrayed by Tom Wilkinson to stop sabotaging an important if highly unethical lawsuit that their firm is defending. In fact, the central crisis of the film is precipitated when Wilkinson's character strips off his clothes in court and announces that he is Shiva, the god of death. The viewer is then informed that Wilkinson's character suffers from bipolar disorder and that he is in the midst of a manic episode. There is also a feeling that the current manic episode stems from a hardened and honest appraisal that Wilkinson's character is conducting regarding his participation in the more ruthless aspects of what is legally allowed by his profession but that he nevertheless has increasingly experienced as ethically highly suspect. In other words, his mania occurs in the context of his life experiences. It does not occur in a vacuum. The causes of his behavior allow for an interpretation of his worsening health. The viewer is thus able to appreciate the fact that his psychiatric symptoms are drawn from the unique social milieu of his particular world.

However, the clearly manic behavior demonstrated in the opening courtroom scene is substantially less subtle than the much more informative and nuanced scene that occurs later in the film. At this point, Clooney's character is trying to convince his psychiatrically suffering law partner to get help. His partner is calm at first, but it takes little for him to veer toward the agitated behavior that is more characteristic of mania. Additionally, he is holding more than a dozen loaves of bread and describes the bread as "the *best* bread" he's ever had. He is not at first behaving in a way that would cause anyone to worry for him, but he becomes more agitated than his circumstances warrant when Clooney's character confronts him. This particular scene allows the film to demonstrate the subtleties of mania as well as the more obviously dramatic aspects of manic episodes.

Michael Clayton is an important film because it allows the viewer to recognize that people with even severe bipolar illness can be extremely high functioning and at the same it emphasizes the damage that can occur if the disease is not properly addressed. In other words, both empathy as well as understanding are fostered by the careful and nuanced portrayal of mania throughout the film. This is a theme that we will continue to come back to over and over throughout this book. *Film creates displacement.* Recall that we defined displacement in the introduction of this book: It is a defense mechanism that allows us to more comfortably and even honestly examine aspects of ourselves that are otherwise difficult to embrace. As it turns out, there is evidence that the more compelling a film happens to be, the greater the extent to which viewers will relate to and be curious about how to help the protagonist (Caputo & Rouner, 2011).

I have used *Michael Clayton* professionally in work I have done with patients who have a hard time reconciling the lack of entirely diminished functioning in the setting of what is still clearly dangerously manic behavior. Mr Wilkinson's character is clearly suffering when he lashes out at Mr Clooney's character. Nevertheless, even within this state, he is able to construct sound and potent legal arguments. His suffering is not demonstrated by his inability to think. His reasoning is very much intact. Rather, his condition is defined by his grandiosity on display in the setting of his utter lack of insight into his outlandish expectations. Individuals with these challenges and perhaps especially their families have found *Michael Clayton* useful when they attempt to reconcile the very high-level functioning of someone who is nevertheless still significantly in danger from the ongoing destructive behavior characteristic of mania.

Interestingly, there are substantially less films that focus on depression despite the fact that depression is a much more common experience among viewers. Approximately 15% of a given population of adults will suffer from depression whereas only 1–3% will suffer from bipolar disorder. This is not due to a prejudice toward depression, but rather through the natural drama that conditions such as mania bring to a story. Depression, with its low energy, poor concentration, and increased feelings of guilt, does not necessarily lend itself as readily to a compelling plot. One might even hypothesize that the overwhelmingly higher number of films featuring mania when compared to depressive symptoms has led the general public to assume that mania is in fact more common. To my knowledge, this has not been formally studied, but it is certainly my experience in teaching with film that even medical students tend to overestimate the amount of bipolar disorder based on the over-representation of this condition in on-screen storytelling. Nevertheless, there are in fact many marvelous films that manage to portray the effects of depression on the person suffering from depression as well as on those around them. Ironically, many of these films are billed as comedies or at least as drama–comedy mixes. Although this has not been directly addressed in the literature, it seems to me that there are two main reasons for the seemingly odd juxtaposition of comedy with the melancholia that characterizes depression. First, to make depression palatable in a dramatic, on-screen format, comedy might help to inject relief from what can otherwise be a drab, off-putting, or pessimistic story despite the best intentions of the storyteller. It is also the case that some of the symptoms of depression itself might seem, in entirely innocent and authentic fashions, to be at least somewhat humorous. The rigidity of depression, coupled with the frequent belief among those who are depressed that that nothing can be done to make matters better, can readily conjure the pacing neurotic characters that directors such as Woody Allen have made famous (Tutt, 1991). However, it is also possible that by making these stories at least somewhat humorous, we connect with the depressed characters in ways that would otherwise seem nearly impossible. Current films that fall into this category include *Its Kind of a Funny Story*, *The Squid and the Whale*, and *Little Miss Sunshine*.

But what about films that do *not* take a comedic approach to depression? The challenge for these stories involves the simultaneous creation of empathy for a condition that many have suffered and at the same time would rather not actively contemplate. People who have been depressed generally might not want to consider how they felt once the depression has lifted. As noted earlier, depression affects roughly 15% of the general population. That number suggests that there is a very high likelihood that those watching on-screen narratives that feature depression will be familiar with the themes of the story through personal experience. These issues make a dramatic and enticing portrayal of depression that much more challenging. The 2009 movie *Helen* is a good example of a film that managed to walk this difficult tightrope. The story involves a successful and much respected professor of music slowly and dangerously drifting into an increasingly dire and suicidal depression.

Helen is notable for the seeming lack of reason offered for the main character's depression. Her own husband notes that he can't understand why she feels so sad. He reminds her of the love that she receives from both family and professional colleagues, and he appears to suggest that her depression makes little sense given how fortunate her life has been. The film in fact received a good deal of press from several major publications precisely because the story resisted offering an interpretable narrative for her depression. "She's not sad," one doctor says to the husband. "She's ill."

To this end, *Helen* speaks to the bewilderment among those who suffer depression as well as to those who try to make sense of why the depression is occurring. Helen's lack of health begs for an explanation, but, as with most cases of clinical depression, there are no clear reasons why she has succumbed to this particular illness. While some viewers might find this kind of ambiguity uncomfortable, many who have written about the film noted that it was exactly the absence of reasons for the depression that creates empathy for Helen. This is not to say that depression itself lacks meaning. The meaning of the illness to the person with depression is not the same as *making sense* of the illness. That message, in and of itself, creates a powerful story, in part because it challenges us to accept the inexplicable and at the same time to remember that the absence of explanation does not necessarily equal futility. (We will come back to these concepts in the final chapter of this book.) Therefore, in ways that are similar to *Michael Clayton*, *Helen* creates empathy and understanding. I have known patients who have taken solace in the paradoxically hopeful message that *Helen* offers, reminding them that even in the absence of understanding the reasons for their depression, there are ample and proven treatment options.

MEDICAL ILLNESSES

Before we discuss the depiction of non-psychiatric illnesses in film, it is important to note that the heading "Medical Illnesses" is a bit of a misnomer. Psychiatric illnesses are by definition also medical illnesses. To separate psychiatric illness from medical illness is to fall prey to the dualism that often stigmatizes psychiatric suffering. Nevertheless, much of the literature exploring these issues in media use the phrase "medical illnesses" and that is the reason the term is used here. It is also the case that virtually every film that focuses on medical suffering has at least some element of emotional suffering as well. The separation of these films into psychiatric and medical categories is thus somewhat artificial. This will become apparent as we move forward with our discussions, but for now it is useful to discuss these topics as separate entities.

A sometimes overlooked but extremely well-regarded film for the purposes of this discussion is the 1985 biographical film *Mask*.

This movie tells the true story of Roy (Rocky) Dennis, a teen born with severe craniofacial dysplasia. This condition is characterized by abnormal facial bone growth that results in a rather striking and often painful appearance. "Craniofacial" simply means that it is primarily the head and the face that are affected, and "dysplasia" is a medical terms for abnormal growth. Eric Stoltz received numerous accolades for his breakout role as Roy, and Cher, playing Roy's mother, was equally celebrated. Briefly, the film follows Roy's coming of age as he relishes his first crush, pushes back against doctor's predictions, and generally enjoys life as best he can. Critical appraisal for the film includes the apt observation that the story is almost "too Hollywood to believe," and yet interviews with Roy's family and friends have shown that the film rarely veers from an accurate depiction of Roy's triumphs and tribulations. Rusty Dennis Mason, Roy's mother, has been forthright in numerous interviews that she was told that her son would die far before adolescence, that he would be severely cognitively impaired, and that his limitations would be debilitating and overwhelming (https://www.chicagotribune.com/news/ct-xpm-1986-05-11-8602030023-story.html).

Nevertheless, Roy is gifted intellectually and creatively, lives well into adolescence, never loses track of his hopes, his aspirations, and his limitations. In fact, he actively incorporates his plans for the future together with an honest appraisal of the challenges he's bound to face, including the near certainty of an untimely and early death. To this end, *Mask* represents the central tenets of resiliency that researchers have noted correlate well with greater wellness, better coping, and ultimately full and satisfying lives even in the setting of severe adversity. Generally speaking, resilience is defined as the ability to accept and to make reasonable, honest, and authentic adjustments in the face of adversity (Schlozman, Groves, & Weisman, 2004). As one might expect, much of the literature exploring resiliency stems from investigations into how individuals cope with medical illness. In *Mask*, Roy knows that others stare at his disfigurement. He is aware when others defend against their discomfort with the way Roy looks by engaging in the reductionism of thinking of Roy as a representation of a rare disease. One of the most enjoyable scenes in the films occurs when a younger and less comfortable clinician treats Roy as little more than a specimen. Roy accepts this clinician's approach with just the right amount of amusement and disdain. After the younger doctor finishes his examination, an older and more experienced physician who has long known Roy engages Roy as a unique individual who has incorporated his illness into his sense of self (https://www.youtube.com/watch?v=fc0uxTiUDrE). To this end, *Mask* is the rare narrative depiction that manages to represent illness with appropriate pathos and honesty and at the same time preserves a sense of hope. The film is itself resilient to the metaphoric sickness that often afflicts movies that attempt an authentic but nevertheless one-sided approach to devastating illnesses. Empathy for Roy comes not from sympathy for his condition, but instead from admiration toward his willingness to accept the fact of his condition and at the same time to relish the life that he has. Multiple studies have shown that empathy toward others stems from the recognition of the differences between the self and the other, and at the same time an appreciation of shared values and aspirations. These goals are aptly obtained by *Mask*.

I first used *Mask* clinically as a tool when I was asked to consult to the pediatric ward regarding a young teen who was dying from widespread osteosarcoma, a malignant cancer of the bone. She seemed to the staff less concerned with her prognosis and more interested in discussing whether she'd be healthy enough to attend her school dance. On paper, her request made perfect sense. She'd been looking forward to the dance, and neither she nor her doctors had anticipated the rapid spread of the cancer. She simply wanted the staff to give her a rough estimate of whether they thought she could safely attend the party. Because she asked the staff about the dance soon after she was told that she had less than a few months to live, the staff felt that she was failing to appreciate the gravity of her circumstances. When I asked her about why she was focused on the dance, her first response was to laugh and to point out that she'd been thinking about high school dances long before she'd known she had cancer. She then grew more wistful and acknowledged that she'd never been in love. "I don't think I love my boyfriend," she confided, "But I'll probably never get to go find out whether I truly love someone the way everyone else does. I just want to spend time with him to see what I can learn."

I found myself tearing up during her conversation and her response was to laugh supportively. "I know this sucks," she admitted. "But I can still enjoy the dance." Her thoughtful reconciliation with her illness and her entirely appropriate adolescent aspirations allowed her to focus on how she could best cope with her predicament. Still, when I tried to make this point to some of the pediatricians, they were uncomfortable. "There are more important things than this dance," one argued. That was when I decided to refer to *Mask* and even to show them scenes from the film. The movement of what had been uncomfortable themes onto a visual narrative format facilitated a discussion that otherwise had been difficult to initiate. This is the power that film can bring to conversations about health and wellness.

As we noted at the start of this chapter, there are ample examples of emotional and physical challenges throughout film and television. Summarizing every health condition as it appears on the screen, or every film that explicitly tells the story of someone with a health concern, is far beyond the scope of this book. Nevertheless, it is useful to mention some conditions for which research has suggested a dearth of sympathy or empathy among the general population. To the extent that these stories can help viewers to be more open-minded toward these conditions, these films have the genuine power to heal and to educate as well as to entertain.

Psychosis is a frequent theme in on-screen entertainment. In this book, we shall define psychosis as a general break from knowing what is real. A person suffering from psychosis might suffer hallucinations or have difficulty thinking clearly and coherently. Other signs of psychosis include paranoid thoughts as well as firmly held beliefs that are clearly not true. However, psychosis is often utilized in film as an explanation for violence and the viewer is therefore openly invited to demonize those suffering from psychotic conditions. This is certainly the case in many horror films and thrillers. Classic and well-regarded films such as *The Texas Chainsaw Massacre, Halloween, The Silence of the Lambs*, and *The Visit* are examples of movies where very psychotic individuals are viewed shallowly, as dangerous, and in entirely negative lights.

Still, not all films fall prey to this damaging storyline. *They Look Like People* creates empathy for a young man who is convinced that he is surrounded by demons. *Martin* is an often overlooked vampire movie where it is never clear whether the protagonist suffers from psychosis or not. Non-horror films that have dealt poignantly and effectively with psychosis include the Oscar winning films *A Beautiful Mind* and *Shine*. The independent film *Angel Baby* tackles the extremely difficult topics of negotiating the dizzying bureaucracy of mental health care for those with schizophrenia, a condition characterized by long-term psychosis, who wish to marry and have children. We will revisit some of these films in our discussions in the final chapter of this book.

Similarly, substance abuse, though common in the general population, is often met with a certain amount of derision in community surveys. The unflinching and thoughtful stories in films such as *Clean and Sober, Leaving Las Vegas, Boogie Nights* and *The Basketball Diaries* (to name only a few) have gone a long ways toward humanizing these otherwise highly stigmatized conditions. Even more impressive are those rarer on-screen stories of sexual paraphilias or abnormal desires. These movies address themes that are understandably immensely challenging to depict openly and sympathetically. *The Woodsman* masterfully creates a complex portrait of a protagonist who is sexually aroused by children and has served prison time for child molestation. *Autofocus* addresses themes of sexual addiction and voyeurism. Both of these films have been celebrated for their sensitive discussions of highly charged subjects.

Perhaps equally challenging and complex are those extremely rare films that feature multifaceted and even sympathetic portrayals of antisocial personality and psychopathy. People with these conditions are unable to recognize or appreciate the rights and needs of others. *We Have to Talk About Kevin* addresses the psychological emptiness that a future school shooter suffers and his family's frustrations in making sense of how best to act toward stopping their son from causing harm to himself or others. *No Country for Old Men* similarly addresses the confusion experienced by a hired assassin who struggles to feel the remorse that others expect of him as he completes his work.

In other words, it is possible for even the most difficult topics to be sympathetically and empathically portrayed in on-screen narratives. The same can be said of many physical conditions that many find challenging to address. *The Fault in Our Stars* tells the story of a romance between two teens with seemingly terminal malignancies. *50-50* humorously and unflinchingly describes the fears and resilience of a young man diagnosed with lymphoma who is informed that there is a 50% change that he will die from his disease. In the 1993 film *Philadelphia*, an attorney with HIV sues his former law firm for discrimination after he is fired for hiding both the facts that he is ill and gay. This fact that the movie was made in 1993 is important; today, the treatment of people with HIV has hugely improved emotionally and socially. One might even argue that the popularity and sensitivity of this film paved the way for our more enlightened treatment of individuals who have contracted the HIV virus as well as greater acceptance of homosexuality (Cartwright, 2016).

So far, we have focused primarily on depictions of specific conditions in film and other forms of on-screen entertainment. However, the experience of being sick, regardless of the cause, can in and of itself provoke a lack of understanding and therefore diminished empathy among those who are ill as well as those who are confronted by others who are convalescing. Long periods of disability caused by severe illness or injury can try the patience of all involved, and there are a number of films that focus on these themes. Again, it is beyond the scope of this book to outline an exhaustive survey of all of the available examples. As we have done with other conditions, we can focus on a single movie as emblematic of the challenges of making films that revolve around these difficult themes. The 2016 Netflix produced film *The Fundamentals of Caring* is a quirky, honest and sometimes quite sad depiction of the challenges of coping with the long-term consequences of Duchenne's muscular dystrophy, a life-long affliction that causes early onset muscle weakness, increasing paralysis and death during young adulthood. Given the severity of this illness, it might seem odd to present the story through a somewhat humorous lens. However, the protagonist's anger at his predicament, coupled with his hired caregiver's emotionally paralyzed state in the setting of a family tragedy, provide the opportunity for humor to serve as a healthy, effective, and honest reaction against what could otherwise be viewed as a film in danger of creating little more than a sense of empty pathos among viewers.

The young man with muscular dystrophy *is* in fact difficult to take care of. The movie therefore allows for an honest examination of the frustrations inherent in suffering from and caring for those with chronic and serious illness. I have found this film useful in my work with transplant patients. As the chief consultant to the pediatric solid organ transplant unit at the hospital where I work, it has been extremely helpful to refer patients to this film and others like it that manage to realistically and but never fatalistically portray long-term medical suffering.

Additionally, there are a number of illnesses that are associated with social derision and even ridicule. These conditions include medical challenges such as fibromyalgia and chronic fatigue syndrome, also called myalgic encephalomyelitis. In fact, some have asserted that both of these illnesses lack evidence for being "true" conditions, arguing that the symptoms are in fact "all in the head." In this sense, these illnesses are doubly stigmatized. People with these conditions have their symptoms dismissed and their troubles are lambasted as somehow representative of chronic complainers with relatively minor issues. In fact, chronic fatigue syndrome has been referred to as the Yuppie disease, suggesting that otherwise healthy white collar individuals simply cannot tolerate the normal discomforts of life. Although this book focuses primarily on narrative on-screen fictions, for these kinds of conditions, well-made documentaries might work better at fostering empathy and understanding. The 2017 documentary film *Unrest* is a painful and yet also affirming story of a PhD candidate at Harvard who developed chronic fatigue syndrome and finds herself increasingly isolated and frustrated by other's perceptions of her illness. Because one of the most difficult aspects of chronic fatigue syndrome is the loneliness that accompanies the isolation inherent in the condition, the fact that a community exists among those who suffer from this illness helps those who feel alone to know that there are those with whom they can connect despite the still relative dismissal of their symptoms in some corners of mainstream medicine. I have used this documentary in teaching medical students to foster a greater understanding of the crippling seclusion that occurs among those with diseases that are poorly accepted by mainstream culture.

Lastly, this chapter would not be complete without noting the power film has in promoting general well-being. As we mentioned in the introduction, film, like all of art, has the capacity to allow escapism and displacement. Numerous studies show that the experience of being shown a compelling story is itself neurobiologically rewarding. The appreciation of stories recruits multiple brain regions in ways that are different from virtually any other circumstance. For everyone who has the cognitive capacity to appreciate stories, there are substantial rewards for taking the time to immerse oneself in an imaginary space (Speer, Reynolds, Swallow, & Zacks, 2009). One can argue that stories themselves, and perhaps especially on-screen stories because of their relative facility for fostering escapism, make our brains literally feel better. It would be absurd for me to suggest specific movies as examples. Because we all have different tastes and preferences, each reader will undoubtedly be able to bring to mind a movie or on-screen series that he or she found rewarding. These rewards are strongly associated with better overall health. Film, as we have stressed, keeps all of us healthy.

Some of these benefits stem from the community that film affords. If one were to read all of the Reddit streams for immensely popular shows such as *Breaking Bad*, *Game of Thrones* or *The Americans*, it would likely take more time than watching these series themselves. The same can be said of informal discussions, either digitally or in person, for popular movies. Multiple studies show that community affiliation is associated with greater immune system protection, less overall illness, and more happiness. This might be even more potent with musical expression than with other forms of art (Fancourt et al., 2016). To the extent that the musical scores of movies are integral to the storytelling of movies themselves, film is uniquely poised to reach an extremely large audience. Think of the celebrated and much recognized scores to movies such as *Star Wars*, *Toy Story*, *Chariots of Fire*, or even the eerie repeating piano sequence in *Halloween*. If one appreciates these pieces of music in the presence of others who do as well, we literally and measurably become healthier. Our stress level goes down and our ability to fight disease increases. Remember that on-screen entertainment is one of the few examples of reliably available, readily inexpensive, and widely consumed forms of art. These artistic expressions therefore foster widespread community connection and thus greater health among individuals and populations.

This communal nature of popular film offers the opportunity to engage in potentially controversial national and even international conversations with greater civility and understanding. *The Crying Game* allowed nuanced conversations around issues of gender identity well before this particular topic had even become part of our civic discourse. *Get Out* provoked discussions of race and privilege through the campy narrative of what on the surface was a straight-forward horror film. *Concussion* allowed a sympathetic and yet honest and unflinching exploration of the risks in American football. Film allows the healing that comes with nuanced discussions and the ability to ask difficult questions.

There are of course more films, more on-screen programs, more diseases and more health-related themes that we have not mentioned. It is likely that by the time this book goes to print there will be new stories produced that continue this trend toward increased acceptance and understanding of all forms of suffering. Film, like all of art, cannot help but to draw from themes that are central to the times in which their stories are told. As long as access to movies and streaming entertainment is available, these stories will remain valuable tools through which we can better understand and teach others about human suffering and resiliency.

2

VIGNETTES DESCRIBING THE THERAPEUTIC UTILITY OF ON-SCREEN ENTERTAINMENT

In the previous chapter, we noted that on-screen entertainment offers opportunities for understanding the many complex experiences that illnesses create for those who are sick as well as for their loved ones. We will now turn to the utilization of on-screen entertainment for real-time therapeutic encounters between clinicians and those for whom they care. Indeed, because of the ample availability of video material from in-office computers, clinicians can now access on-screen scenes for treatment as the usefulness of these scenes becomes evident throughout each session with the individual seeking help. This kind of accessibility was not possible as recently as a few decades ago. It stands to reason, therefore, that the use of popular scenes from movies or television programming in therapeutic settings is an emerging field and in dire need of more research. Still, these opportunities show great promise for ongoing and future clinical encounters. As with the previous chapter, we will focus on the use of film for the treatment for specific problems. Once again, because I am physician, the vignettes we discuss will have a necessarily medical flavor. This is not to say, however, that the same processes cannot be used outside of the doctor's office. Finally, as is the case with any attempt to utilize the appreciation of art for healthcare purposes, new examples will arise as further content is created and becomes available.

As perhaps makes sense, examples of specific scenes written about in the treatment literature or mentioned by practicing clinicians tend to focus more often on emotional challenges. Psychological themes by their very nature feature prominently in virtually every story. We will therefore start by discussing particular psychiatric conditions. Furthermore, I will present multiple vignettes that span different diagnoses and different developmental stages. It is important to note that these vignettes are amalgams of many different people. I have taken great care to de-identify the features in each story to protect confidentiality.

SIMPLE PHOBIAS

Simple phobias are defined as discretely and intensely experienced fears that are directly and knowingly a response to specific triggers. For an anxiety reaction to meet the criteria for a simple phobia, the individual must suffer some loss of function as a result of the phobic response. In other words, a simple fear of bridges isn't really a problem in Las Vegas where bridges themselves are in short supply. However, someone with a fear of bridges in the San Francisco metropolitan area might drive literally hundreds of miles out of his way to avoid crossing one of the many bridges that dot the city and its surroundings. Similarly, a fear of snakes isn't a problem in Ireland, but would be highly problematic in a many of the cities in Central America. In each of these examples, the mainline non-medication treatments are exposure and response. Individuals are exposed to the fear-inducing stimuli in increasingly poignant circumstances and taught how to control the increased heart rate and rapid breathing that occurs when the stimuli are experienced. In other words, individuals are trained to recognize when their pulse and respiratory rates are increasing and they are given specific techniques to control these fear responses. If we return to the problem of bridge phobias, an individual might first be asked to visualize a small bridge, then shown an image of a small bridge in a photo or on a computer. At the same time, the individual is helped to engage in already practiced relaxation exercises. Larger and more imposing bridges are viewed and eventually actually visited, and the individual uses the same response extinction techniques once these techniques have been successful with each preceding phobic provocation (Böhnlein et al., 2020).

There are of course multiple online examples of films that meet the needs of exposure for simple phobias. *Sneakers* features and in-depth investigation of the bridges in the San Francisco Bay Area. *Snakes on a Plane* offers more than its share of legless reptiles. However, it is also important that the film or film clips utilized be appropriate for the age of the person in the office. Remember that some might go home and watch the film entirely, despite instructions from their clinicians to pace themselves. This is why it is imperative that parents *and* those asking for help be made aware of the treatment plan and that careful consideration be given to which films are chosen. There may be on-screen entertainment that some find objectionable, and introducing this material without first getting permission from patients and guardians is can cause significant damage.

Let's use a pathologic fear of spiders for our case example. Current epidemiologic estimates suggest that arachnophobia, the fancy word for intense spider fear, is one of the most common simple phobias, present in roughly 3–6% of the global population. The average age of onset of arachnophobia is hard to gauge, but most estimates place it between four and nine years old (Schmitt & Müri, 2009). This means that for most individuals, the on-screen exposure must be carefully chosen. The giant spider in *The Hobbit* is potentially far too graphic for a young child. Fortunately, there exists at least one film that is perfect for this particular phobia when it presents in younger children, as the following vignette demonstrates.

SIMPLE PHOBIA – VIGNETTE

Sara is a six-year-old girl who is brought to a therapist by her parents after she uncovered a nest of spiders in her garage. The spider had laid her recently hatched eggs at the end of the previous summer in the corner of the garage where Sara had stored a box of her favorite dolls and toys. She had forgotten all about these dolls during the winter, but the promise of spring had brought her back to collect her outdoor playthings, only to discover hundreds of tiny spiders crawling all over her beloved toys. She screamed, kicked the box over on its side, and since that day has become severely panicked whenever her family encounters cobwebs or forested areas where one might reasonably expect to find spiders present.

Because of Sara's age, the therapist opted to start with the clips on line of the 1973 animated film version of *Charlotte's Web*. Charlotte, the spider in this particular story, is kind, caring, and connected. Still, she has all the characteristics of a spider – she has eight legs, an intricate web, and she deposits her eggs just before she expires. She also shows her friendliness by writing words of greeting using her web-spinning prowess, and she even utilizes this ability to communicate with others to save Wilbur the pig from being butchered. Sara had not seen this film, and her parents granted permission for the clip of the film to be viewed in therapy and also at home. The scene where Charlotte's children greet Wilbur was especially appealing Sara. The baby spiders are sweet and not at all threatening. Sara watched the scene over and over in the office and then again at home. Although she initially felt some fear when seeing this scene, gradually her fear diminished. The therapist then moved to videos of actual spiders, all the while using the relaxation techniques learned in therapy to control her response. Soon, her phobia disappeared altogether.

Traumatic Bullying

Understanding and preventing bullying has received special attention over the last two decades. The rise of the Internet in general and social media in particular has made the effects of bullying more potently experienced and less likely to dissipate. As a result, there has been a well-documented increase in traumatic reactions to bullying, whether the bullying takes place in person or over the Internet. The new digital world seems to amplify the effects of bullying and at the same makes prevention efforts particularly challenging. In addition, the ongoing and more publicized prevalence of bullying has made themes concerning the effects of bullying increasingly central to on-screen storytelling (Yahn, 2012).

However, in order to address the growing emotional challenges associated with both bullying behavior and among those who are on the receiving end of these kinds of assaults, a careful and nuanced approach to understanding the factors leading to as well as the effects of bullying is necessary. Most researchers agree that bullying involves repeated physical or psychological attacks from a person or group of people who deem themselves more powerful than the ones that they are attacking. Researchers also note that in any bullying scenario there are essentially three equally important groups who make bullying possible: the person or persons who are doing the bullying, the person or persons who are being bullied, and the bystanders. All three of these entities play important roles in the enactment of bullying activities. Clinicians will encounter individuals in need of help from each of these groups, and a comprehensive public health effort to stop bullying will require ample attention to all who are involved. It is also the case that many members of each of these groups often change. Those who bully have been bullied. Those on the sidelines are likely at some to be involved, either voluntarily or by coercion or attack. To this end, it is imperative that clinicians develop an appreciation for the ways that these all of these groups interact. Bullies, those who are themselves bullied, and individuals on the side lines all have been shown to experience increased difficulties with anxiety, depression, substance abuse, post-traumatic stress disorder, and non-specific traumatic reactions (Obermann, 2011).

Despite ample attention to the problems created by bullying, schools and communities have had a difficult time containing these behaviors. In fact, bullying scenarios and their downstream costs to health and well-being have been steadily increasing. A very large study conducted nearly two decades ago in the Journal of the American Medical Association found that nearly 30% of students in American grades 6–10 (approximately age 12–15 years) had experienced some involvement in bullying behavior. Among those students, 13% had engaged in bullying behavior, nearly 11% had themselves been bullied, and just over 6% reported that they had both bullied and been bullied (Nansel et al., 2001). The Center for Disease Control and Prevention (CDC)'s Youth Risk Behavior Surveillance System found that roughly 20% of youth in American grades 9–12 (approximately 14–18 years old) report being bullied on school property (Stopbullying.gov). In addition, although bullying seems to cluster among early- to mid-adolescence, adults also suffer the effects of bullying. Studies have found that adults who feel bullied more often report that the experience occurs in the digital realm. A Swedish study found that nearly 10% of just over 3,000 surveyed individuals reported being bullied over the Internet in the previous six months (Forssell, 2016). Again, as a result of the increase in bullying across age, socioeconomic, and international populations, stories involving bullying are prevalent in movies and on-screen serials. This suggests that clinicians can use these stories to better understand those who have experienced bullying as well as those who have participated in bullying. On-screen stories explicitly involving bullying include Netflix's *13 Reasons Why, Bandslam, Mean Girls, Carrie,* and *Swimming with Sharks.*

The challenge in using stories from the increasing repertoire of movies that feature bullying as a central theme is the relative one-sided nature of the storytelling. In *13 Reasons Why,* for example, those who have done the bullying are depicted relatively concretely rather than with any real nuance. However, those in need of healthcare support for their involvement in bullying do best when they can appreciate and empathize with all of the players in the complex bullying dynamic. The following example demonstrates how one can use a specific scene that is readily available online in helping a young person who has been the victim of bullying.

TRAUMATIC BULLYING – VIGNETTE

Michael is a 13-year-old boy who skipped a year of school and is therefore a freshman at the local public high school. Although he is gifted intellectually, his voice is still high-pitched and he is shorter than many of his peers. As a result, he is quickly labeled a "dork" and "a loser" by students in his own class. At one point he is tripped in the locker-room in his physical education class, and he remembers viscerally the experience of rising to his feet in front of his locker where someone had used a sharpie to draw male genitals and written the word "dork" in large letters. The entire scene was captured on multiple smart phone videos and passed quickly through the hallways of the school.

As Michael became aware of his notoriety, he started refusing to come to school. Eventually, the school became aware of the perpetrators of the prank and the video slowly disappeared. The students who had participated in the prank were disciplined, and the school held a mandatory assembly stressing their zero-tolerance policy for bullying of any kind. For Michael, however, the damage was done. He suffered nightmares, headaches, decreased appetite, and his grades faltered. His emotional state became paradoxically worse when one of the persons who had tripped him sincerely wanted to apologize. The individual texted Michael, tried to stop him in the hallway, and even paid a personal visit to Michael's home. Michael refused to meet with the apologizing student, and eventually Michael was himself suspended for pushing a student in the school cafeteria.

Michael's clinician felt that for Michael to recover, he would need to appreciate the possibility that the apology was sincere, that the person who had tripped him had himself likely been bullied in the past, and that offering the apology was in fact an act of respect and even courage. However, Michael could not address these issues. He simply could not imagine any good coming from the student who had harmed him, and he continued his slow, downward spiral. The clinician then elected to utilize a clip from the popular 1999 television show *Freaks and Geeks*. In the particular scene, an older and somewhat intellectually insecure student engages in what is at first a tentative and then later a heartfelt détente with a group of boys he had previously relentlessly ridiculed and bullied. In the final scene, the older student, played by James Franco, joins the younger students for a game of *Dungeons and Dragons* and genuinely enjoys himself. When Franco's character objects to be assigned the role of a dwarf, the younger boys tell him that dwarves can do things that non-dwarves cannot. The message, it seems, is clear. Everyone brings both talents and liabilities to the table. As the game progresses, Franco smiles more, jokes with the other teens, and implicitly apologizes for the way he has treated the boys. The younger boys in turn slowly embrace their new relationship with this once menacing older student. Although they do not become close friends, they grow to respect each other and each side feels better as a result (https://www.youtube.com/watch?v=hJAGxAeV7YU&t=188s).

When Michael noted that the story seemed "too stupid to be true," the clinician agreed. "It's Hollywood," the clinician admitted. "The scene might have happened too easily, but the feelings could still be real." Discussing this scene led Michael to accept the apology of the student who had tripped him and eventually to embrace and be proud of his role as the youngest student at the school.

Autism Spectrum Disorders

In 2013, the American Psychiatric Association removed Asperger's disorder from its list of diagnoses. Instead, individuals who had relatively normal language development but lacked the ability to detect social cues (the main characteristic of what had previously been considered Asperger's syndrome) were coded as having high functioning autism, and diagnosed under the larger umbrella of autism spectrum disorders. It is beyond the scope of this book to detail the reasons for this change in terminology, but generally speaking the intent was to ensure services for those persons, most often children and young adults, who had normal language development but still suffered substantially due to their social confusion and misreading of cultural cues (Kite, Gullifer, & Tyson, 2013). Some heralded these changes as creating new opportunities for those who had previously been left without a stronger argument for accommodations and treatment. Others felt that this created a somewhat misleading number regarding the prevalence of autism and related conditions in the United States and throughout the world. It is certainly the case that the rates of autism have steadily and dramatically risen. According to the CDC's Autism and Developmental Disabilities Monitoring Network, autism spectrum disorders were estimated to affect about one in 59 children throughout the United States in 2014 (https://www.cdc.gov/mmwr/volumes/67/ss/ss6706a1.htm#suggestedcitation). Since then, current data suggest that the number continues to rise. Similarly, studies overseas have found that between 1% and 2% of individuals suffer from autism. Given the increased numbers of diagnoses as well as the frequency of media interest and front-line coverage, it is no surprise that characters with autism spectrum disorders have become increasingly common in works of fiction, including movies and television programs. Critics have also noted that previous depictions of autism, such as Dustin Hoffman's role in *Rain Man*, have given way to more accurate characterizations of the syndrome of autism and its accompanying challenges. Hoffman's character possessed preternatural talents with math and numbers, a condition called Savant Syndrome, as well as a particularly odd way of relating to the world. Some have wondered whether *Rain Man* led some to feel that Savant Syndrome, present in only 1% of those with autism, was in fact a common feature of the illness (https://www.theguardian.com/commentisfree/2018/dec/17/rain-man-myth-autistic-people-dustin-hoffman-savant). However, more recent characters with autism include Brick on the American program *The Middle*, Sheldon on *The Big Bang Theory,* Sam on the comedy-drama *Atypical,* and the central character in the South Korean and later the American version of *The Good Doctor*. Sesame Street has even introduced a puppet who has been diagnosed with autism spectrum disorder. As more and more stories incorporate increasingly realistic portrayals of this syndrome, many have wondered whether previously held biases against autistic individuals have been affected. A 2019 study among college students found that watching one episode of *The Good Doctor* resulted in a more accurate and less prejudiced view of autism than a lecture containing the same information (Stern & Barnes, 2019).

This study suggests that movie and television portrayals can also help individuals with autism to better understand and cope with their capabilities and challenges. The following case uses the 2009 film *Adam* as a tool for helping a teen boy to accept when and where he needs to ask for and accept help in navigating his day to day life.

AUTISM SPECTRUM DISORDERS – VIGNETTE

Will is a 16-year-old boy who has recently moved and although previously home-schooled, now attends a local secondary school. Recently, he has started to resist schoolwork because "no one understands" him. He notes that he will try to make jokes with other class-mates or flirt with girls in the hallways but that his initiatives are either ignored or taunted. He also has a hard time understanding assignments as they are explained in class, and though he is quite bright, his answers to questions in English and History classes are often marked poorly as too concrete and lacking in nuance. His teachers are flummoxed, given his higher than average vocabulary, and his parents note that previous pediatric visits have suggested that his mannerisms are somewhat odd but that he is otherwise healthy.

Will's therapist diagnoses him with autism spectrum disorder and asks Will, his parents and his teachers to help Will to become more comfortable in asking for clarification regarding assignments and even interpersonal interactions. This helps somewhat, but Will remains frustrated that he is unable to connect with peers, and he often fails to understand humorous quips that are traded in the hallways and outside of class. He feels lonely and isolated, though he is unsure how to remedy this. Will's clinician asks that Will and his family watch the 2009 film *Adam*, a romantic drama about a young man with high functioning autism who has learned to ask others for clarifications when he is confused by routine occurrences and is at the same time bluntly and sometimes uncomfortably hon-est with friends and even romantic interests. Adam practices telling those to whom he is close that he has Asperger's syndrome, a diag-nosis that Will is aware would have applied to him were it not for the recent change in terminology. As a result, Will is able to view an appealing and on-screen template for how to interact with others. He starts bringing jokes home and asking his parents and his thera-pist the meaning of the punch-lines. He literally learns the social cues that he understands come naturally for others, and he credits *Adam* for helping him to accept responsibility for these challenges.

Non-psychiatric Challenges

Non-psychiatric illnesses have always featured prominently in film. To the extent that stories in all formats document the crises that are common throughout life, it stands to reason that on-screen narratives would frequently portray medical illnesses of all sorts.

Some movies focus on life-changing injuries. For example, the 2011 film *Soul Surfer* documents the true story of a professional surfer who lost her arm following a near fatal shark attack. Similarly, the extremely popular American television program *Friday Night Lights* spends a good amount of time following the ways that the once star athlete copes after he is paralyzed from injuries sustained in an American football game. Other stories focus on grappling with chronic or potentially fatal illnesses. *The Fault in Our Stars*, *50-50*, and *Love and Other Drugs* are all examples that feature the challenges of severe illnesses as central to the fundamental storyline. It is beyond the reach of this book to detail all of the on-screen stories that use medical illnesses as part of the narrative arc. An excellent review can be found in an article in the *Annals of Internal Medicine* that also summarizes the success of the film *Lorenzo's Oil* (Jones, 2000).

Clinicians have often utilized these movies to increase empathy among students and the general public, but less commonly in overtly therapeutic settings. Indeed, while clinical literature is ripe with examples of using film for psychological and psychiatric treatment, there are virtually no case reports or studies documenting the therapeutic utility of movies themselves in treating non-psychiatric illnesses. To some extent, this makes sense. One can tell a story about the meaning of cancer or liver dysfunction, but it is arguably more often the case that the desire to explore meaning as a therapeutic exercise takes place in the mental health clinician's office. Nevertheless, as we have already stressed, this creates a false distinction. Psychological adjustment is a necessary element to coping and resiliency in the face of medical disease. Any movie about medical illness in theory could be utilized by healthcare providers in the service of helping patients and their families to cope with their illnesses.

MEDICAL ILLNESS – VIGNETTE

Nancy is a 36-year-old woman who's second child, a girl named Sharon, was born with severe spinal bifida and subsequent paralysis. She feels ill-equipped to handle the challenges of raising what she has been told will be a severely disabled daughter. Her husband travels often for work and for her family to afford the help that Sharon requires, it is not possible for him to change his occupation or his work schedule. As a result, Nancy becomes increasingly anxious, obsessional, and unable to sleep. She worries about how Sharon will ever cope in the "real world" and she feels helpless and hopeless when she contemplates Sharon's future. She also has started to neglect the needs of her older child, a three-year-old boy, who has become increasingly frustrated with the lack of attention and subsequently suffers frequent and severe tantrums. Sharon's pediatrician finds that Nancy seems unable to tolerate even a conversation about plans for Sharon's future, but she also steadfastly refuses referral to a therapist, stating that "it wouldn't do any good." In passing during one of these visits, the pediatrician mentioned that "plenty of children" do very well despite serious disabilities. The pediatrician had in fact recently watched *My Left Foot*, the Oscar winning film about a boy who can move only his left foot but does so with gusto and enthusiasm. The pediatrician asks that Nancy and her husband watch the film. Although they were reluctant, both parents agree and find the movie inspiring, although they admit that they had wrongly expected that the film would confirm their fears about their daughter's future. The overwhelmingly positive regard for the film among critics and the general public leads Nancy to re-evaluate her worries about Sharon's disabilities and provokes her to enter therapy to focus on how best to handle her anxieties while attending to both of her children.

Changes Throughout the Life Cycle

As we have noted, in addition to understanding and caring for those with illnesses, the maintenance of health requires a nuanced understanding of the needs of individuals across different developmental stages. Illnesses will look different at different stages of the life cycle, and to this end, films can help us to understand the tribulations that are characteristic at different ages and at different stages of maturity. Because the changes during childhood and adolescence are so steep, films are especially useful for exploring these formative years. There are countless coming of age films and television programs, and indeed entire books have been devoted to this particular genre of film. Some have noted that coming of age movies are not in fact representative of how true adolescence takes place. After all, critics note, many older high school students move freely among the different cliques that movies like *Mean Girls* or *The Breakfast Club* have made famous. In fact, Gil Noam and others have pointed out that the formation of exclusive and therefore exclusionary groups is particularly and normally a phenomena that takes place just after the start of adolescence. Children between the ages of approximately 11 and 15 more often coalesce into small groups. Noam (1999) has coined this developmental pattern the Psychology of Belonging. Healthy development has therefore been conceptualized as increasing comfort with moving out of specific and exclusive groups and moving instead among different groups. Multiple studies have noted that happy and well-adjusted teens are accepted across a wide swath of groups, reflecting their willingness to express their multiple and sometimes even paradoxical interests. The "goth" boy who is also a celebrated athlete is a bit of a cliché, but this example is also indicative of what most developmental specialists would agree is a sign of emotional stability and comfort with one's own identity formation.

This means that films often portray the ways adults recall high school and earlier as opposed to actual representations of the current secondary school experience. Movies like *The Breakfast Club, Sixteen Candles, Super Bad*, and *Ladybird* might all fall into this category of film. On the other hand, some films show normal developmental crises that occur in the setting of severe stress. The protagonist in *Perks of Being a Wallflower* appears to suffer from depression and trauma, but his difficulties are seen through the lens of other relatively well-adjusted teens. It is, therefore, arguably the rare film that accurately portrays normal adolescence in the absence of any psychological or medical challenges. This is in part due to the necessary tension to tell stories themselves. If there are no challenges to be overcome, and if those challenges are not to some extent novel to the viewer, then the film runs the risk of being hackneyed or boring. In this light, films like *Eighth Grade* and *Booksmart* feel that much more remarkable. The girl in *Eighth Grade* has lost her mother to illness, and it is clear that some of the central tension in the story is created by her father's attempts to help his daughter to manage the rocky and uncomfortable road through early puberty. However, most of her challenges are in fact tied to the simple challenges of getting older. Even Bo Burnham, the film's creator, worried that the awkwardness of the film would feel too real to viewers (https://www.hollywoodreporter.com/features/making-eighth-grade-how-bo-burnham-brought-his-anxiety-screen-1162239). However, the film was instead hailed as a critical and heartwarming, if also cringe-worthy, artistic success. Similarly, *Booksmart* tells the story of two girls who assume they have been ostracized for their attention to academics throughout high school. The girls and therefore the audience are delighted to find that contrary to what they've been led to believe, the two protagonists are welcomed with open arms as school draws to a close and the end of the year parties commence.

Because so much of adolescence and early adulthood is tied to identity formation, coming of age films more and more often feature characters who are representative of our diverse population. The recent remake of *A Wrinkle in Time* featured a protagonist with an African-American mother and a white father. Although the fact that she was neither black nor white played a minimal role in the plot, many viewers and especially viewers with similar ethnic backgrounds to the protagonist were particularly moved precisely because the story did not hinge on race. It felt normalizing to these viewers to see themselves represented in a film whose plots did not specifically revolve around issues of ethnicity (https://ew.com/movies/2018/03/07/reese-witherspoon-wrinkle-in-time).

Often, understanding the world through the eyes of children and teens is a challenge for parents and other caregivers. Some have wondered whether memories of coming of age are themselves too painful, and that as a result some adults steadfastly refuse to put themselves in adolescent shoes. Regardless of the reasons, this difficulty represents an ideal opportunity for film to create empathy in a therapeutic setting. Because therapeutic work with children and teens inevitably involves increasing the understanding of their caregivers regarding the challenges that young people encounter, one can utilize popular film to help parents and teens to better understand one another.

CHALLENGES DURING ADOLESCENCE – VIGNETTES

Bill is a 12-year-old boy who has become more isolative over the last five months since the start of middle school. His best friend has become a gifted rugby player and has expressed little interest in spending time with Bill after school. This change in after school activities represents a major departure for Bill from how most of his early school had progressed. Although Bill does not meet the criteria for depression, he does harbor the conviction that no one at the school would want to be his friend, and he prefers instead to come straight home at the end of the day to watch endless You-Tube videos. His parents are particularly frustrated with his seeming social stagnation and seek the advice of a therapist to whom they had been referred by Bill's pediatrician. "This can happen at the start of middle school or high school," the therapist notes, and recommends finding new activities for Bill to participate in where he can meet new friends. His parents, however, are reluctant. Why can't he just meet new friends without their help, his parents wonder. After all, Bill's friendship with the boy who was now preferring to play rugby after school had formed organically and with minimal parental effort. The parents are worried that if they help Bill with this challenge, Bill would miss the valuable opportunities afforded by finding activities and friends on his own. The therapist suggested that the parents watch *Eighth Grade* to gain an understanding of the changing emotional and developmental landscape of early adolescence when compared to elementary school. His parents agree, and because they find the film's depiction of the protagonist's challenges difficult, they wonder about the psychological accuracy of the film. The therapist assures the parents that the film is accurate and that most teens require some kind of support through this difficult developmental period. However, Bill's parents continue to have a difficult time accepting that the difficulties faced by the protagonist in eighth grade as consistent with normal developmental challenges. The therapist therefore refers the parents to multiple critical appraisals of the film's accuracy. Once the parents accept that Bill's challenges are both normal and in need of some parental intervention, Bill, his parents and the therapist are able to devise specific plans to help Bill to better integrate with his peer group.

So far, we have focused primarily on challenges faced both in sickness and health of children and teens. However, there are of course countless films that explicitly explore challenges faced by adults, including their struggles with their own developmental issues. Well-conceived romantic comedies such as *Juliet Naked, High Fidelity, Love, Actually,* and *The Goodbye Girl* are all examples of these kinds of explorations. Issues such as relationship stagnation, infidelity, whether or not to marry and how one knows whether one is in fact in love (and what the phrase "in love" even means) are all central components to these movies. As the developmental scholar Erik Erikson noted, if adolescence involves crises of identity, then early adulthood is more concerned with crises of intimacy. In other words, it is necessary to know who you are before you can understand whether you love someone.

Other films have admirably tackled the motivations and fears of adults entering middle age. These movies can be jarring even if they simultaneously allow one to smile from time to time. *Nebraska* explores a middle aged man's relationship with his angry and aging father. *Osage County* and *This is where I Leave You* explore family dysfunction and at the same time offer recipes for familial reconciliation.

An entire sub-genre of film explores the difficulties that occur when adults must care for sick spouses or parents. *Still Alice* focuses on the relationship of an older woman as she struggles to cope with her dementia and her children feel increasingly powerless to stop the progression of her illness. *Terms of Endearment* explores the conflicted feelings that a middle aged couple experiences when their far-from-perfect marriage is interrupted by the wife's diagnosis with late stage cancer.

Many clinicians have remarked that one of the hardest aspects of therapeutic work is helping others to see how their behavior is of itself causing much of the presenting distress. This is perhaps especially the case when adults behave in maladaptive ways around their children, even if those same patterns of behavior are success-ful and rewarded outside of their parental lives. The following vignette uses the movie adaptation of the French stage-play *God of Carnage* into the on screen film *Carnage*.

MALADAPTIVE PARENTAL BEHAVIOR – VIGNETTE

A local middle school asks the school therapist to meet with par-ents who have become extremely belligerent during educational meetings intended to formulate a plan for how best to accommo-date their son's severe dyslexia. Their 12-year-old child Edward often feels lost in school and as a result has missed a good deal of learning from not being able to complete the reading assign-ments or the in-class reading exercises. His self-esteem suffers at least as much as his grades despite the school's good-faith efforts to meet Edward's academic and social needs. School officials feel strongly that they have conducted a thorough assessment of how best to teach Edward, including a district sponsored reading spe-cialist hired as an outside tutor as well as instituting changes in the ways that teachers interact with Edward so that Edward will be less likely to feel ashamed of his difficulties. However, Edward's parents, both highly successful and well-regarded litigators, come to each meeting prepared to argue with school officials for more services. They even instruct their son not to follow the recommen-dations of school officials for fear that compliance with these regu-lations would constitute agreement with the existing practices and thus negate the possibility of future additions to the educational accommodations. When the therapist asks the parents why they want more services, the parents seem indignant. "He's our son," the mother said. "It's our job to fight for the most possible." At this point, the therapist asks the parents to explain more about how litigation works, and the therapist was impressed by the similarities to litigation practices and the rigidity of the parents in the educa-tional meeting. "What works in the courtroom won't always work here," the therapist notes, but the father objects, pointing out that the school meetings were "adversarial in nature," just as a court proceeding could be. At this point, the therapist asks the parents to watch *Carnage* before their next meeting the following week.

A charitable interpretation of this bitingly sardonic film involves two well-meaning couples who meet to resolve mounting tensions after their young children are involved in a playground fight. Each has the best of intentions, but to some extent they thwart any attempt at an amicable resolution by enacting the skills that have served them well outside of their roles as parents. The therapist is clear with the parents that the movie is extreme, and that he did not see the parents themselves as similar to the parents in the film, except to the extent that the parents felt stuck as they each tried to use the skill set that they most valued in a circumstance where the skills themselves seemed highly unlikely to be successful. Edward's parents return to the next meeting with school officials and explicitly note that they will drop their litigating stance and instead work toward a compromise more consistent with what the school can offer. In this instance, they noted that the film, while clearly exaggerated to stress the ways that adults can lose track of the methods by which they achieve their goals, had helped them to imagine how the school might be experiencing their belligerence.

This chapter demonstrates the ways that film can foster empathy and understanding in therapeutic settings. Whether one considers formal psychological or medical diagnoses, or a better understanding of the general challenges that we encounter throughout the life-cycle, the near endless supply of on-screen entertainment offers countless opportunities to help others to appreciate more adaptive ways of thinking or behaving. To that end, one can literally prescribe a film. I certainly do. However, as each of these vignettes demonstrates, there are a number of important caveats. Although this may sound obvious, one should always watch a film or television program before "prescribing it." I have met clinicians who have heard others suggest the use of a specific film in therapeutic settings and have therefore recommended these films to patients despite never having seen the movies. This runs the risk of miscommunication and broken alliances with patients who feel as if an assignment were given despite the clinician him or herself not having engaged in the same assignment. Second, it is highly unlikely that a given on-screen story will exactly match the issues that a clinician wishes to illustrate to a patient. It is therefore advisable that clinicians tell their patients about why this particular film came to mind in the treatment, how the clinician hopes the film can be helpful, and where the film might notably veer from what the clinician is trying to convey. Finally, if patients are reluctant to watch a film, it should never be forced. Required viewings run the risk of empathic failure. Instead, let the individual know why the film might be useful, in what ways the film might also fall short, and stress that if one is not interested in watching the film that the treatment will of course continue. An alternative can involve watching clips of the film during the appointment. This keeps the treatment within the boundaries of the office and allows the clinician to choose the issues on which he or she wishes to concentrate the therapeutic energy.

However, one of the many wonderful things about art is the fact that it has therapeutic utility even in the absence of a formal therapeutic engagement with a clinician. The next chapter will focus on how one can use film on one's own to foster greater health, well-being, and a more powerful and compelling sense of community.

3

THE HEALTH BENEFITS OF COMMUNITY ENGAGEMENT IN FILM

Film has the power to create cohesion and a greater sense of community and belonging. Importantly, these qualities can also lead to alienation and even feelings of exclusion. Again, this makes sense when we remember that film is, among many things, a potent form of artistic expression. Art can unite and art can also be divisive. Some may feel that a work of art speaks very personally and positively to their own experience. By the same token, others who have perhaps not had the same experiences or do not agree with the light in which a given experience is expressed, might feel personally but negatively affected by the same film. However, a central premise of this book is that film derives its power from its immensely varied stories, coupled with its unparalleled ease of accessibility. In short, there is a film for everyone and for all convictions. What appeals to one person may not appeal to someone else, but the breadth of film engenders its ability to provide a sense of understanding and empathy among and within a wide swath of audiences.

These qualities are further enhanced by the tendency for works of popular culture other than film to be frequently adapted for movies or television programs. Books, both fiction and non-fiction, have been adapted for the screen since the beginning of the motion picture industry itself. There exist conflicting reports of the first novels adapted for film, but among those mentioned include George Melies' *Gulliver's Travels* in 1901 and *Robinson Crusoe* in 1902. Before that, a single 45-second scene called *Trilby and Little Billie* was reportedly created from the best-selling 1895 novel *Trilby*. Unfortunately, there are no surviving copies of this film and records of the cast and the crew have been lost. However, in both cases it is worth noting that the books chosen already enjoyed huge popularity. Early filmmakers reasoned that if already popular books could garner large and loyal fans, then the movie versions of these stories would produce similar outcomes. For the purposes of this particular book, these historical observations suggest that film has long been appreciated for its capacity to appeal to entire communities. Although the results of these efforts were not immediate, eventually the process of transferring the written word onto the screen appealed not just to the fans of the original stories, but also to a new group of enthusiasts who preferred for a variety of reasons this visual form of storytelling. Interestingly, this process has not earned universal acceptance from the story-tellers themselves. When the contemporary author Dennis Lehane was asked about his work toward adopting his story *Mystic River* for the screen, he famously quipped that comparing books to movies was like comparing "apples to giraffes."

Nevertheless, it is hard to deny that these kinds of comparisons happen as frequently in academic journals as they do in more pedestrian settings like dorm rooms and dinner parties. Any cursory exploration of online discussion forums demonstrates that there are always those who are eager to discuss both forms of storytelling, and often the discussions involve comparing the books to the movies. Furthermore, these discussions frequently revolve around what form of storytelling is preferred. To this end, the presence of popular stories as film adaptations creates cohesion among enthusiasts of both the written word and on-screen narratives. Indeed, as the forms of storytelling continue to diversify through video games and podcasts, these narratives too find their way to the screen. The *Resident Evil, Halo, Tomb Raider* and *Final Fantasy* video game franchises are just a few examples of video games that have successfully yielded multiple movies. More recently, popular audio podcasts such as *Homecoming, Limetown* and *Dirty John* have all been produced for streaming entertainment. The ability for almost all forms of storytelling to readily lend themselves to on-screen depictions helps add to the wide spread sense of community that film engenders.

The scholarly literature detailing the unique ability of film to foster community cohesion is as rich and varied as film itself. There are history papers that note the effects film can have as a potent tool of propaganda during both war and peace. During World War II, the German film industry produced multiple courtroom dramas that depicted the new laws under the Third Reich as fair and just (Drexler, 2001). During the same time period, films produced by Allied nations were similarly laden with rousing affirmations of their own war effort. The fact that film has been utilized as part of an effort to build community support for both sides of the conflict speaks to the power of film to convey a message, and that to some extent, the nature of the message matters less than the quality and sophistication of the storytelling. Thus, as film production became more advanced, one could argue that it became similarly more sophisticated as a uniting or a divisive source. In the United States, perhaps the most notorious example of this process is D. W. Griffith's 1915 silent film, *The Birth of a Nation*. This was by far the most technologically advanced film of its time, and it gained popularity in part because of the extent to which the novel on which it was based, Thomas Dixon, Jr's *The Clansman,* was already well-known. Although the film clearly depicted an overtly racist political agenda, it was also celebrated for its technical prowess. The overall story of the success of *The Birth of a Nation,* despite its off-putting ideology to many, serves as a warning that opinions can be swayed both explicitly and subtly through well-made video productions. The ability of film to unite is therefore potent regardless of the message around which its unifying power centers. This unique feature of on-screen storytelling explains the history of film as a cohesive force as much as it makes plain the reasons that films are even today both criticized and celebrated as propaganda. Community cohesion happens throughout a given ideological spectrum, and these varied notions are all thus well represented in film and television. Although this book has so far primarily focused on fictional or non-fiction narrative films, much of the literature around film's cohesive power has been described through the potent reach of well-made documentaries. There are thousands of documentaries that have conveyed clear and successful rallying cries. Scholars have written about the ability of documentaries to convey information that unites communities amidst potentially polarizing concepts inherent in discussions of race and economic status (Bell, 2018). Secondary school students in the United States have created documentaries as a means of better understanding and relating to the history of their surrounding environment (Morris, 2018).

Nevertheless, the cohesive power of film goes far beyond the world of documentaries. There are studies noting the power of cinema to bring together worlds as esoteric as the LGTBQ community in twenty-first century Israel (Padva, 2011), and as wide spread as the universal appeal of the Star Wars and Harry Power franchises among children and adults. In fact, communities themselves have noted that simply viewing film together can create community cohesion, regardless of the films themselves. There are community film festivals in towns as small as Niagara Falls (advertised as the smallest international film festival in the world) and in cities as large as Berlin, New York, and Cannes. Virtually all who are asked the purpose of film festivals answer with some version of what Victor Leschenko, the organizer of the Ukrainian Film Festival Docudays, replied when he was asked to describe the impact of community film festivals in current times. "It's sharing," he replied. "Film Festivals are helping at the frontline of an increasingly polarized world" (https://www.screendaily.com/comment/whats-the-purpose-of-film-festivals-in-the-21st-century/5108598.article).

However, this is a good time to recall that this is a book about the role of film as it relates to *health*. The discussion of film and its power to create community therefore begs an important question. *To what extent is fostering community related to improved overall health and well-being?* Numerous studies have documented the beneficial health effects of community cohesion. These studies involve epidemiological investigations, neurobiological observations, and even hormonally based evidence for the power of community as a protective force. In all cases, if we accept the power of film to create communities of similarly interested individuals, then we can comfortably make the case that the appreciation of the art of film and television has the power to make us happier and indeed healthier.

From an epidemiological perspective, neighborhoods that are more aesthetically pleasing and intact demonstrate greater overall health (Henderson, Child, Moore, Moore, & Kaczynski, 2016). Communities that spend time together at gatherings such as group singing also do better from a health perspective (Pearce, Launay, Machin, & Dunbar, 2016). Intriguingly, many communities have found that they experience greater cohesion when they enjoy the opportunity to view films together. The small town of Oakley, Kansas in the United States noted this when it opted to devote special resources toward keeping its local movie theater open (Benet, Grout, & Dagostino, 2009). Similar findings were realized on a much larger scale in Istanbul, Turkey when local citizens developed grassroots movements to rescue historic movie houses (Yasar, 2019).

Neurobiological observations have shown that community cohesion precipitated by connection through language and ritual is characterized by greater overall mental and physical health. For humans, it neuroanatomically feels good and reduces stress to connect with others. This is demonstrated through findings such as the fact that lower levels of post-traumatic stress disorder (PTSD) have been documented in similar communities that have greater social cohesion than in those without (Johns et al., 2012). Because the cause of PTSD involves heightened exposure and response to external stressors, one can reason that communities that are more united are less prone to the effects of stress on overall brain function. This finding is even more fascinating when one notes that people who watch movies, and especially humorous movies, experience lower overall levels of stress in general (Khamsi, 2005). In this light, movie-watching is beneficial through its effects on community cohesion as well as for individual health and well-being.

All of this suggests that popular movies and television programs, through their capacity to decrease stress and increase community engagement, are potent facilitators of health. It stands to reason that the more popular a given film or television program, the greater its capacity to be quite literally good for all of us. Also, popularity need not be measured in terms of numbers. Even small groups of devoted fans for cult favorites will benefit from the community that film engenders. Consider the impact of television programs like *Game of Thrones* or *Downton Abbey*. While these showed aired, there were weekly watch parties, online and in-person discussions, critical and popular press expositions about each episode and social media networks devoted to connecting like-minded fans. If anything, those who enjoy less well-known genres benefit even more from the tendency of fans to gather together. There are similarly devoted groups invested entirely in B-grade horror films or the early projects of the cult-film director John Waters (Webster, 2012).

In fact, people of all ages and of all tastes gather to enjoy the art that film has to offer. It's a genuine joy to watch the local opening of any much loved on-screen story. Children line up in costume to see the Harry Potter movies. Whole dinner parties revolved around the *Downton Abbey* movie. New friendships were forged and old friendships were further solidified. This is the power of film to heal and to make healthy.

HOW TO CREATE COMMUNITY AROUND FILM

We have established that the creation of community is good for our health. These communities decrease stress and increase our overall well-being. There is even evidence that community cohesion is immune-protective. Researchers at Britain's Royal College of Music have documented that communities that gather together to enjoy or to participate in musical performance experience an increase in immune-protective cells that help to fight infection in those undergoing treatment for cancer (Fancourt et al., 2016).

But how can one create these communities? If this book is to make the case that our overall health stands to benefits when we gather together to enjoy film, then we must also discuss the most efficient means by which we can reap these benefits. In fact, current concerns about decreasing community involvement in multiple domains has generated interest in researching the best methods to re-establish community, including the communities that revolve around on-screen entertainment.

One of the ironies of this body of research is its implication of social media as a potent reason for the dissolution of diverse communities, but its simultaneous endorsement of social media as an important tool toward the development of community cohesion even among seemingly diverse populations. Thus, while some studies note that the tightknit and ideologically rigid world of social media gatherings can make others feel unwanted or even threatened, there exist competing observations that the potential for social connection, including social connection around film or television, is made easier through the ease of social media utilization. Rural communities, for example, have noted that Facebook groups allow otherwise disconnected farmers to gather either online or in-person for discussions of a favorite movie. Researchers have investigated the cohesive and beneficial effects of online ratings for film and television. Studies have also shown that social media gatherings have the power to eliminate racial bias in both the choice and the appreciation of on-screen entertainment (Weaver & Frampton, 2019). There have even been investigations into the benefits of social media in helping artists to gather in the creation of film itself (Scarnato, 2018).

All of this suggests that one of the most potent ways to enjoy the community health benefits of film is to utilize the strength and reach of online communications. However, one need not turn only to social media to locate communities that gather because of a shared interest in film and other forms of on-screen entertainment. Libraries and communities across the world now regularly host screenings and subsequent discussions of popular on-screen entertainment. The Alfred P Sloane Foundation's Science on the Screen program pairs feature films shown at independent theaters with noted scientists and scholars as discussants (https://scienceon-screen.org). The Science on the Screen program started at a single theater outside of Boston and has over the last decade spread to dozens of theaters in both large and small towns across the United States.

4

HEALTH BENEFITS OF
INDIVIDUAL ENGAGEMENT
WITH FILM

In Chapter 2, we focused on the means by which clinicians can utilize on-screen entertainment in their efforts to help those individuals who seek their help. However, individuals themselves may find movies or television programs useful in helping their clinicians to better understand their dilemmas. One of the first documentations of this technique involved the use of closed circuit television in psychiatric facilities in the 1950s. A 1957 article in the *Archives of Psychiatry and Neurology* found that when the staff at inpatient facilities curated the television that was available for inpatient entertainment, the patients themselves often chose specific programs to discuss with their clinicians (Tucker, Lewis, Martin, & Over, 1957). This is of course a much more rigid and, at least by today's standards, overly paternalistic approach to helping patients to be comfortable using video entertainment as part of their treatment. It is also the case that the choices of on-screen venues and stories is much more varied than it was in the earlier days of television. The time and effort necessary to curate today's media options makes this approach impractical as well as improper by today's standards.

However, people often mention movies to their clinicians in all fields of health, and to some extent, the effectiveness of this means of therapeutic communication has been under-studied and under-reported. One explanation for this lack of scholarly investigation might be the already general acceptance and ubiquity of this practice. It makes sense that those wishing to help clinicians to better understand their plights would turn to popular media as a means of expressing the various feelings generated as a result of the clinician's attention. These references also serve as an efficient method to allow clinicians to better understand how those they seek to help are feeling regardless of the state of their treatment. To be clear, this happens in all fields of medicine. The famous rectal exam scene in *Fletch* was mentioned by at least ¾ of the patients on whom I performed a digital prostate exploration during my medical training. The scene is humorous but also deliberately uncomfortable and therefore captures in a lighthearted way the discomfort that patients experience when this particular aspect of the general medical examination takes place (https://www.youtube.com/watch?v=9-zf2UBp7fY). Similarly, I've had colleagues mention to me that patients have asked them to watch *The Doctor* (1991), presumably to convey their anxieties following a frightening diagnosis or as they prepare themselves to undergo a surgical procedure. Some argue that patients use film to efficiently convey what they worry will be otherwise difficult to succinctly and clearly state during an office or hospital visit.

Given the at least anecdotal frequency of this practice, it is important for clinicians to keep in mind the general rules of therapeutic engagement. All discussions with patients during a therapeutic encounter should be in the service of the patient. This might seem obvious, but the introduction of a popular film into a treatment setting could lead clinicians to fall into the familiar mode of discussing a film with their patients in the same manner as they would outside of the bounds of a clinical engagement. Simple questions such as "what was it about this film that you liked," or "why do you find this television program important" are helpful inquiries toward protecting therapeutic boundaries. Patients have their own agendas with the films they wish to discuss and it is important for the clinician to avoid hijacking that agenda with their own opinions of the merit of the film itself.

A PATIENT RECOMMENDS A FILM TO
HIS PSYCHIATRIST – VIGNETTE

A 35-year-old man kept mentioning the romantic comedy *You've Got Mail* to his psychiatrist. The psychiatrist had not seen the film, and she was not particularly interested in watching it. She did not tell her patient that she did not wish to see the film, but it became apparent during patient visits that it was important to the patient that she sees the film before they could continue. After consultation with colleagues about managing her own resentment at engaging in a "leisure activity" as part of her treatment for her patient, the psychiatrist decided to watch the movie. At the next visit, her patient asked her whether she had seen the film, and when she told him that she had, the patient began to cry. This was not what the psychiatrist had expected, and she asked the patient what he was thinking. The patient noted that he needed the psychiatrist to see the film so that he could explain to her his guilt at imagining what it would be like for him were his wife to succumb to her cancer and die. "I'd be the good guy," he said. "Just like Tom Hanks. No one would blame someone like me for wanting to meet other women...." He then went on to describe the troubles that had existed in the marriage and his guilt and shame over sometimes wishing that his wife were no longer alive so that he could make new romantic connections with social and emotional impunity. The psychiatrist helped the patient to feel more comfortable discussing these issues and reassured him that the desires to explore new romantic interests were common issues in many marriages, and she referred the patient and his spouse for couples' therapy. In this instance, what seemed on the surface to be a relatively straightforward romantic comedy had become a source of identification and shame for the patient. The patient was clear that he needed the psychiatrist to watch the film to facilitate these extremely difficult discussions.

Using Film for Health and Well-being Outside
of the Clinician's Office

Increasingly, researchers have noted that engaging with film and other forms of on-screen entertainment carries therapeutic benefits outside of overtly therapeutic settings. Dr Gary Solomon, a psychologist who has written frequently about the health benefits of film, notes that films allow viewers to experience emotions that they might otherwise have a hard time acknowledging (https://www.webmd.com/mental-health/features/movie-therapy-using-movies-for-mental-health#1). To be fair, this assessment is potentially flawed. According to Dr Solomon's conclusions, movies by definition can therefore derive their benefit *only* if the viewer wishes to experience these otherwise sequestered emotions. However, much of psychotherapy as well as current interests in mindfulness and greater self-awareness is predicated on the fundamental premise that people *feel* better when they are able to safely experience difficult emotions. Furthermore, we have already made the case that on-screen entertainment is immersive, allowing the viewer to undergo a kind of hypnotic experience. If the protagonist is upset, the viewer might feel similarly upset. Many argue that viewers will not allow themselves to feel what they truly do not wish to feel, similar to conclusions that researchers have long believed regarding susceptibility to hypnosis. To this end, the burgeoning literature supporting the stress relieving properties of enjoying movies and television programs appears to be best explained by the cathartic experience that we discussed earlier in this book.

Interestingly, the beneficial effects of movies appear regardless of the genre of movie that is enjoyed. What seems to be most important is that the film itself is enjoyed by the viewer. Thus, there are studies showing decreased emotional tension following comedies, tragedies, and even horror films. With regard to horror films, scientists have tied the appreciation for frightening movies to the thrill one feels after riding a roller-coaster. Others have noted that viewing multiple movies has the potential to substantially improve vocabulary and overall learning (Webb, 2010). Some have even postulated that thrillers and horror films allow us to better understand our less savory feelings and urges and to reckon more honestly with these feelings, thus allowing for decreased overall cortisol levels (https://www.youtube.com/watch?v=WoYrpA3v-38; Strizhakova & Krcmar, 2007). Similarly, investigators have long been aware of the paradoxical enjoyment viewers experience when they watch a sad movie (Schramm & Wirth, 2007). The idea that sad stories are themselves helpful is hardly novel. The natural philosopher David Hume noted that after experiencing sadness people often have a greater appreciation for art and beauty (Oliver, 1993). Still, the breadth of sad or otherwise off-putting movies from which to choose demands more investigations into the best methods by which viewers can utilize movies to enhance their health.

In fact, there exists a somewhat competing body of research noting the deleterious health effects of movies and television. Problems such as obesity and isolation have been tied to the ample availability of home entertainment and the obviously stationary state in which most on-screen media is consumed. Others have noted that sexually aggressive behavior is heightened by graphically violent movies with sexual themes (Huesmann, 2007), and there have been case series of PTSD documented in children for whom the triggering traumatic event is viewing an unsettling movie or television program (Bozzuto, 1975). These caveats accentuate that the recommendation that individuals simply watch more films to relieve stress and improve health is naïve and oversimplified. Movies must be developmentally and emotionally appropriate to incur a therapeutic benefit. Not all movies will carry the same or any therapeutic benefit for different viewers. Furthermore, if one watches nothing but movies for hours and hours, whatever cardiovascular risk that is decreased by the resulting decrease in stress hormones is clearly offset the medical dangers of extreme physical inactivity. Using films as rewards for engaging in exercise or even viewing films during exercise are viable methods for alleviating the risks of inaction with the enjoyment of film.

In addition, in some cases, engagement with film confers unequivocally negative health effects. Some forms of on-screen story telling portray struggles with poor health in a rather negative light. For example, films that are despairing with regard to the possibility of help for those with suicidal thoughts are more likely to make viewers feel more hopeless about their own predicaments. This is especially this case among adolescent viewers who are already suffering from suicidal feelings (Till, Tran, Voracek, Sonneck, & Niederkrotenthaler, 2014). In these instances, however, the same films could still be viewed as empathic. The stories do in fact reflect what the viewer is thinking and feeling, but the effects of engaging with these films is deleterious and some would argue even dangerous. The most recent widespread example of this is the Netflix franchise *13 Reasons Why* (Carmichael & Whitley, 2018).

As one might expect, much of the effects of engaging in film are tied to the context in which the film or television program is viewed. Movies that negatively portray illness could be used positively if one is using these films to illustrate the persistence of stigma. On the other hand, if the agenda in watching a film is to demonstrate that the lack of belief in the very presence of certain illnesses – this is sometimes the case with the ways that psychiatric illnesses are portrayed – then the deleterious societal effects of this message can be uncomfortably supported. Films such as *Split* or *Primal Fear* could have this effect. As all indications suggest that offerings of a wide variety of on-screen entertainment will continue to grow, research will need to focus on how best to take advantage of the beneficial aspects of film and at the same time how best to mitigate risk.

5

TECHNIQUES FOR HEALTHCARE PROFESSIONALS TO UTILIZE FILM

In Chapter 2, we discussed specific examples in which healthcare professionals use film as part of their therapeutic endeavors. In this section, we will expand on these ideas by examining the research in support of the utilization of film in the service of health care apart from individual treatment. As we noted, there exists a good deal of anecdotal evidence in support of these practices. However, there is also a growing body of research in support of these ideas. Generally speaking, research supports using film for public education, professional education, and treatment.

THE USE OF FILM FOR PUBLIC EDUCATION

Advertising and sponsorship in on-screen entertainment are potent tools of public health engagement. Much of the data in support of these practices comes from what public health officials ask filmmakers to censor rather than on what content they are asked to include. For example, there have been numerous efforts to curtail the sponsorship through advertisements of nicotine and alcohol in films themselves. Importantly, these efforts have not focused on the content of the films, but rather on the commercial advertisements that appear during breaks in the story or as product placements within the story (Millett, Polansky, & Glantz, 2011). Also, it is interesting to note that although many of these efforts were first enacted in more developed nations decades ago, ongoing attempts to decrease these kinds of commercial endorsements have now moved to the developing world and are showing measurable results (Unknown Author, 2016).

These findings have happened in concert with a similar body of knowledge showing that the behaviors in film that are associated with poor health also carry the potential for deleterious effects among vulnerable viewers. Movies where smoking either nicotine or illicit substances among teenagers and adults is present increases the likelihood that young people will engage in these same deleterious habits. There exists evidence as well that when the content of films or television programs features other unhealthy behaviors, those who see these films are similarly at risk. Examples include violent behavior, abuse, and self-harm. As with smoking, these risks seem most pronounced among age-related vulnerable populations – teens and young adults who are more impulsive and prone to peer pressures (Huesmann, 2007).

Indeed, one can argue that these effects are increasing as the power of parental censorship of movies and television continues to decrease with the spread of online entertainment options. It is not as if behaviors that are associated with poor health are new to film – what has changed dramatically is the diminished ability for adults to be aware of the media that younger populations are viewing. In addition, there is an important set of alternative explanations for these increases. It isn't only access to potentially objectionable or inappropriate material that has risen. As we have made clear, the breadth of what can be watched has also become richly varied and detailed. One needs, therefore, to guard against a knee-jerk response that all of what we watch has negative public health consequences. It is possible that for some viewers, the irony and satire in programs like *The End of the F***g World* are realized and have the potential therefore to be experienced as neutral or even beneficial. After all, the escapist nature of on-screen entertainment allows the very benefits that we celebrated in earlier chapters of this book. If viewers can watch programing with these benefits in mind, consciously or not, then they will vicariously explore the behaviors, including the negative consequences of these behaviors, without actually enacting them once the program has ended.

This brings up an interesting set of questions. If on-screen entertainment has the power to provoke both negative and positive health-related activities, how can we know which individuals are vulnerable and which stand to benefit? In some cases, the answers to this inquiry are relatively straightforward. Already suicidal viewers will feel more suicidal when they view a movie with mental health nihilism (Till, Tran, Voracek, Sonneck, & Niederkrotenthaler, 2014). There are numerous studies in support of these caveats. However, we also know that people who are feeling sad will sometimes feel better even after watching a tragic story (Larsen, McGraw, & Cacioppo, 2001). This suggests that vulnerability must be carefully evaluated and for the present time is best assessed on a person by person basis. None of this, however, answers an even more fundamental question: *Are there any films that one can reliably use with universally good public health outcomes?*

This last question is not new. The ABC *After School Specials* of the late 70s and early 80s were an attempt to create savvy and yet clearly agenda-driven health-related stories. Researchers have argued that these programs, literally airing on TV around the times that American teens were getting home from school, deliberately and productively portrayed adolescents as having the wisdom and autonomy to make healthy choices (Elman, 2010). However, others have noted the mixed messages that many of these programs espoused. Feminist researchers have suggested that the frequent presence of Tomboys and more "masculine" girls were presented both as anxiety-provoking as well as accepted by other characters in these dramas (Pike, 2011). The message, according to these critics, seemed to be that it was OK for girls to be a little masculine, but that there was also a threshold after which the masculinity would become abnormal. It is therefore possible that there were unintended negative health effects from these programs. Others have more outwardly decried what they saw as an overt agenda to wrongfully normalize potent social issues such as teen pregnancy, alcoholism, and drug abuse (Amanda Renee Keeler, 2016). As with any popular cultural phenomenon, conclusions about these kinds of programs are difficult to consistently draw and often fraught with the biases that viewers and researchers bring to the subject matter regardless of the content on the screen. Because gender dysphoria, early pregnancy and substance abuse are all clearly themes of public health interests, it is important that these early attempts at public health mass media outreach be carefully scrutinized.

ABC's *Schoolhouse Rock* is another initiative that sought to capitalize in an entertainment format to educate children in America about grammar, math, spelling, and history. Because facilitated mastery of these fundamental subjects helped students to excel in school and to therefore experience less stress and overall increased self-esteem, it is entirely reasonable to view these endeavors as having a public health benefit. Most adults who were raised in America between 1973 and 1985 still fondly remember these 5–10 minutes interludes of the *School House Rock* short films that aired on ABC in between the ritualized viewing of Saturday morning cartoons. Indeed, entire generations learned the preamble to the United States Constitution by humming the words to the music it was set to on one of the more popular segments (Calvert & Tart, 1993). Unlike the After School Specials, *Schoolhouse Rock* was overtly didactic and did not feature a narrative story. Instead, folk-rock music was independently composed and matched to important topics. Some historians have even noted that teachers as ancient as Plato and Socrates felt that the use of music was a necessary component to learn new material, though when one considers the origins of the Schoolhouse Rock concept, it seems doubtful that the executives at ABC had such lofty aspirations. The ABC television network did not in fact pay for these highly produced animated shorts without considerable government pressure. In the early- and mid-1970s, all of the major American networks were under fire by congress to reverse what some worried was the growing presence of violent and adult content in mainstream television. *Schoolhouse Rock* was an attempt to deflect some of this criticism. In fact, current researchers have pointed out that there were slightly subversive messages to the *Schoolhouse Rock* history curricula. Episodes describing the American Revolution accurately showed slaves and other disenfranchised members of colonial society as central to the revolutionary efforts (Ovetz, 2011). While this is certainly consistent with the history of the American Revolution, these depictions were not always consistent with what was at the time being taught in US classrooms. It is possible that some students were therefore met with resistance to what they had been taught from the content of *Schoolhouse Rock* and therefore experienced more rather than less stress from these commercial educational endeavors.

In addition to on-screen programs and movies with overt public health or public education agendas, researchers have noted that there are specific aspects of filmmaking that make this form of artistic expression ideal for public health research and outreach. One very large study sought to discover what particular qualities of films themselves most effectively contribute toward public health efforts. After evaluating over 3,000 articles, the authors of this study determined that film allows unique cultural perspectives to be easily accessed by the target audience, leading to more seamless participation in public health initiatives and greater opportunities for advocacy. In other words, the very qualities that make film so accessible are those that allow film to operate as a potent public health tool (Baumann, Merante, Folb, & Burke, 2020).

Finally, movies and television programs can be utilized as potent public health messages even if this is not the intended use of the film itself. The Science on the Screen Programs sponsored by the Alfred P Sloan Foundation has used films such as *Night of the Living Dead* to discuss the spread of contagions, *Medicine Man* to stress the need that we preserve natural habitats because of the possibility these habitats hold for new medical discoveries, and *GATTACA* to discuss the pros and cons regarding our increasing understanding of what our genetic codes can predict about who we are and what we can achieve (https://scienceonscreen.org). In all three of these films, thematic elements were paired with a speaker versed in the relevant public health inquiries that these themes bring to the forefront.

To some extent, the use of films to illustrate public health issues are governed by the dramatic elements that certain health issues disproportionately bring to the screen. A study for the *Journal of General Internal Medicine* found that the most common diseases featured in films were psychiatric, followed by neurologic diseases, alcohol dependence, and infectious diseases. This study noted in fact a relative dearth of films featuring oncologic diseases and cardiovascular diseases, despite the high numbers of these illnesses in the general population. This finding, therefore, suggests that public health messaging from feature films might highlight some illnesses in ways that are not consistent with the actual burden of the health challenge (Perciaccante et al., 2019).

This is similar to the earlier observation made in Chapter 3 that there are more films about mania than depression, despite the fact that the number of people with depression in the general population is substantially high than the number of people who suffer from mania. Any attempt to use feature films or television programs as a means of starting a public health discussion should take into consideration and openly address these population imbalances.

FILM FOR PROFESSIONAL HEALTH CARE EDUCATION

Clinicians and educators have long used the power of film to teach virtually all aspects of health education. *Academic Psychiatry*, a leading medical education journal, has an entire section devoted to the use of media in psychiatric teaching. I have had the pleasure of serving as the associate editor of this section for the last five years. Articles have discussed the developmental tribulations of adolescence through the lens of Buffy the Vampire Slayer (Schlozman, 2000), the diagnostic queries presented in Star Wars (Hall & Friedman, 2015) and Super Hero Movies (Taylor Williams, 2012) and whether the titular character in *Napoleon Dynamite* suffers from Asperger's syndrome (Levin & Schlozman, 2006). The 2016 keynote address at the Association for Academic Psychiatry conference, an international meeting devoted to psychiatric education, utilized a scene of syncope from the movie *Stand By Me*, a well portrayed hypomanic episode from *Silver Lining Playbook*, and the doctor–patient interaction in *Mask* as examples of the ways one can use film in teaching psychiatry. During my tenure as an adjunct instructor at the Harvard Graduate School of Education, I turned to the films *Ordinary People* and *Welcome to the Dollhouse* for both didactic and assessment purposes among graduate level students studying to become school counselors. Indeed, given the fact that new films and programs are constantly being made, there is no shortage of available material. Recently, for example, the Disney film *Frozen* (Hickey, 2018) has been used to teach different forms of psychotherapy. One could argue that the fact that stories are themselves reflective of the human condition, movies can be viewed as ideal vehicles for psychiatric educational exercises. Once again, the immediacy of film makes this form of art ideally suited for discussion in pedagogic settings, and perhaps especially in mental health education.

Importantly, these ideas have been studied qualitatively and quantitatively. As with many of the topics in this book, entire curricula are based on what we will attempt to summarize in this single sub-chapter. Inevitably, readers will recall and subsequently discover new examples of this growing body of research. Some of the most recent findings include a study that looked for movies that medical students might watch on their own to further familiarize themselves with pertinent medical themes. Rather than start with the films themselves, the authors of this study looked at the World Health Organisation's Global Burden of Disease Survey and then chose movies that best reflect the questions provoked by these particular illnesses. *Trainspotting* was chosen for its focus on substance abuse-related psychosocial determinants of health, *Ordinary People* for its discussion of trauma, suicide and family dynamics, and *Rachel Getting Married* for its portrayal of the guilt and shame inherent in anxiety, depression, and substance dependence (Wilson, Heath, Heath, Gallagher, & Huthwaite, 2014). Others have studied the use of movies to teach the nuances of medical ethics to medical students and residents in medicine, and there are even investigations into the act of making films themselves as a means of better educating healthcare workers about difficult issues (Nam, Cha, & Sung, 2019).

However, not all are in favor of this practice. Some have argued that the limited available time for healthcare education makes the use of film less time-efficient. Others have noted that humanities professors are better suited to teach film than healthcare workers, and that using film in healthcare education therefore shortchanges both the critical appraisal of film as well as what the healthcare educator could offer in the absence of using films in the first place. One study showed that students learned as much from films as they did from a more traditional lecture, and that the films took more time (Bhagar, 2005). In some ways, the contradictory nature of these investigations might have more to do with the teachers themselves than with the technique of using film for healthcare educational purposes. If an instructor is comfortable and confident with this kind of teaching, then the lesson itself seems more likely to be successful. However, if an instructor who would prefer not to use film is forced to do so but would otherwise have delivered the same teaching without the use of cinema, then the teaching is most likely best accomplished in the absence of the utilization of film in the classroom. This is consistent with research suggesting that the emotional engagement of the teacher is a key determinant of the extent to which successful teaching takes place (Kinner & Belmont, 1993).

Because psychiatric and psychosocial themes are more commonly featured in movies, it is possible that films themselves are more often used in psychiatric education. Still, there are ample examples of the use of film in healthcare education to teach stigma reduction and even to help students to better grasp the day-to-day struggles of many non-psychiatric medical challenges. A film that approaches both of these issues is the 2012 Drama *The Sessions*, a film that helped viewers to understand the limitations and libidinal urges of individuals suffering from paralysis (Marini, 2016). Other studies have looked at the changing depictions of physicians through cinema and used these changes to help medical students to better understand the reception they can expect when they start to practice medicine. According to an exhaustive examination of films covering eight decades, both the kinds of medicine depicted on screen and the portrayals of the doctors themselves have substantially changed over time. Doctors are portrayed more often in either surgical suites actively operating on their patients or in a more active role with patients, in both instances with patients portrayed as passive recipients of the doctor's interventions and advice. This study also noted that while depictions of physicians were mostly positive through the 1960s and 1970s, starting in the 1980s doctors were increasingly more likely to be portrayed as paternalistic, aggressive, and arrogant (Flores, 2004). Again, because film often represents prevailing societal views, these kinds of investigations can help future and current doctors to change the ways they practice medicine in order to more completely meet the emotional needs of their patients.

Finally, healthcare education through films and on-screen entertainment need not be limited to discussions of medical practice or even to depictions of specific illnesses. Film can also be used to generate inquiries into potentially thornier issues in health care. Throughout medicine, there are ongoing debates around how one best defines normality. These kinds of discussions involve an intricate interplay of psychological and age-appropriate descriptions as well as existing and no longer accepted societal norms. It might be difficult for students to understand that homosexuality was for a very long time considered in and of itself a disease. However, one study noted the positive influence of overtly gay characters on shows such as *Will and Grace* as major influencers of more positive views of gay and lesbian behavior in mainstream media (Battles & Hilton-Morrow, 2002). Similarly, movies like the 2008 film *Milk* start with archival footage of police raiding gay bars, following laws that were in part made possible by the medical establishment's willingness to declare homosexuality a dangerous disease despite a lack of compelling evidence for such strongly held views. In this way, movies can help students to grapple with the possibility that there are currently designated diseases that will cease to be considered illnesses as societal changes take place.

In all instances, discussions of film in the service of medical education should be kept non-judgmental. Open-ended questions as straightforward as "what was watching that scene like for your," or "do you find this scene realistic" are good ways to allow a discussion to organically take shape. Instructors should also guard against their own nostalgia. The emotional salience that film can create might lead teachers to believe that a movie or television program will be more warmly received by students than students who are unfamiliar with the film will understand. If an instructor uses an older film that is dated or even likely to be unfamiliar to most of the students, it is a good practice to describe the contents of the film in the context of both the goals that the instructor has in showing the film and in explaining material in the film itself that current viewers might misread or even find objectionable. The following case example from my own experience teaching medical students illustrates these important aspects of using film in educational efforts.

THE USE OF AN ICONIC TELEVISION SCENE TO TEACH
BASIC ASPECTS OF ADOLESCENCE – VIGNETTE

In teaching about the unique qualities of adolescent brain development and its subsequent effects on adolescent behavior, an episode from the critically acclaimed American television show *Freaks and Geeks* was shown to medical students. The scene, set in the mid-1980s in a middle class American household, features Nick (played by Jason Segal) serenading his romantic interest Lindsay (played by Linda Cardellini) to the classic 1980s' slow rock ballad *Lady* by Styx. In the scene, Nick invites Lindsay to his house after both he and Lindsay realize that Nick's parents will not be at home. Nick invites Lindsay to the basement where he has lit dozens of candles and asks Lindsay to sit down as part of what he envisions will be a grand romantic gesture. Although some might argue that Nick's actions are based in a rather mature understanding of the power of an intensely authentic chivalric act, many viewers, myself among them, view this scene as cringe-worthy (https://www.youtube.com/watch?v=ZzrMrglib6c). The first time I used this scene, some students were bothered by what seemed to be on overly aggressive approach by Nick and at the same time an overly acquiescent reception by Lindsay. In the current and long-overdue climate of concerns regarding sexual aggression, I realized that I had to change my approach to mention that at the time, this behavior was not considered "stalky" (as one student put it) but instead a misplaced show of affections. As I continued to refine my use of this scene, I started instead to explain the scene first as if it was a real case and not a scene from a television show. I didn't tell the students that what would follow would be on an on-screen display of what I was presenting as a case example. Instead, I showed the students a series of slides summarizing the scene as if these were a patient description. I described a 17-year-old boy inviting a teen girl to his house, forcing her to listen to him sing, and then gently pushing her down next to him so that they could cuddle on the couch. The differential diagnosis of this kind of behavior was subsequently discussed, including mania, borderline personality disorder, pathological stalking, and even some neuropsychiatric conditions such as Huntington's disease. Students were then shown the clip from the episode and asked whether any of these diagnoses still made sense. Inevitably, there was laughter as well as an admission that someone (and usually more than one student) felt that they had been in either Nick or Lindsay's position in their own lives. In other words, the scene became more familiar and more normalized. In this fashion, by increasingly refining the use of what had otherwise been a rather dated and potentially objectionable television scene, we were able to discuss normal adolescence and to address the ways that societal expectations for adolescents have continued to change.

Empirical Evidence for the Use of Film by Healthcare Professionals in Therapeutic Settings

In Chapter 2, we discussed specific films useful in individual treatment. Despite the rather common practice of healthcare practitioners in all disciplines at least anecdotally using on-screen entertainment for therapeutic purposes, there is surprisingly little literature documenting the effectiveness of these techniques. This might be because the use of a given movie is uniquely personal to both the person receiving care and to the caregiver, thus making standardization of this practice difficult and therefore challenging to study. Another explanation is the close relationships between themes common to on-screen storytelling and similar narratives of everyday life. Perhaps studies looking at the use of film of television are rare precisely because a discussion of something as common as film or television, arguably the most available and consumed forms of art and popular culture, happen so naturally in therapeutic encounters that it becomes impossible to separate the use of film from the everyday occurrences in healthcare delivery. In other words, we are always talking about movies and television programs whether we are in the doctor's office or our own living rooms. Although this second premise might at first seem outlandish, think of how often any healthcare encounter has begun with "small talk" about commonly experienced events like much-watched streaming serials or which of that year's Oscar nominations have been seen. If we believe that no conversation happens by accident, then it stands to reason that some of the alliance of health care derives from the common experience of shared popular culture. The author and scholar Francis Kaplan wrote numerous articles and books arguing exactly this commonality. Nevertheless, many riders have to create the lack of empirical evidence for these practices, and some have worried that the practice of actually assigning films for therapy runs the risk of placing the practitioners needs over those seeking help. This is of course more likely in psychotherapy, but theoretically the risk could occur in all fields of medicine.

The exception to this relative lack of evidence concerns the use of popular media as distractors during difficult procedures. Dentists often use and have studied the use of children's programing during dental work (Jayakaran, Rekha, Annamalai, Baghkomeh, & Sharmin, 2017). Additionally, most hospitals, at least in developed nations, use television to alleviate boredom both in the emergency ward and on the hospital floor. Streamed video clips have been used to ease anesthesia induction, to distract during painful procedures such as blood draws, and as rewards for tolerating medical discomfort (Kerimoglu, Neuman, Paul, Stefanov, & Twersky, 2013).

Given the evidence for on-screen entertainment decreasing stress, lowering cortisol, and contributing to health, it is possible that these practices are actively therapeutic in addition to being merely distracting.

There is also a wide breadth of literature that looks at the advantages of films specifically created to help patients to cope with difficult decision and to more accurately give informed consent (van Agt, Korfage, & Essink-Bot, 2014). These studies note that the techniques of filmmaking enhance the overall understanding of difficult topics by patients who are further compromised by the stress of illness. As we have already noted, there are also studies noting that clinicians ought to be aware of the negative influence of film when providing health care. This has been shown for aggressive behaviors as well as for problems such as eating disorders (Koushiou, Nicolaou, & Karekla, 2018). Similar concerns have been raised about increased access to adult film content on the Internet (Duffy, Dawson, & das Nair, 2016), as well as to the already mentioned problem of commercial product placement. To the extent that clinicians can be aware of movie, television, and internet trends that are consumed by mass audiences, they will be better able to guard against these influences among their patients (Linn, 2003).

ON-SCREEN NEGATIVE HEALTH BEHAVIOR EMULATED BY A VULNERABLE TEENAGER – VIGNETTE

A 17-year boy was referred to his pediatrician by school officials after he was caught dealing cocaine at his high school. The pediatrician was asked whether the student had symptoms of substance abuse or dependence and whether these symptoms, if present, could explain his apparent lack of regard for the seriousness of what he had done. The pediatrician did not find that the patient had had any evidence for self-drug use and was concerned that the patient's seeming lack of concern was worrisome for future antisocial behavior. The pediatrician therefore referred the teen to a local psychologist who found that the teen had become enamored of the extremely popular television programs *Breaking Bad*, *Narcos*, and the miniseries *Mad Dogs*. Even though all of these programs did not feature pleasant endings for their antiheros, the teen noted that the shows were clear about where each antihero had made mistakes leading to their eventual downfall. He also noted that these shows had provoked him to research "more successful" real life drug dealers, and he discovered that if they put their money "off-shore" they were able to serve only a few years in prison and to reclaim their money upon release. In this instance, the boy did not show signs of antisocial tendencies so much as a misinterpretation of the exaggerated romance and excitement inherent in the shows he watched. He then conducted his research through the lens of his already present biases. Helping the teen to better understand the downstream effects of his own drug dealing, as well as appreciating the fact that his business acumen was in fact impressive, allowed him to restructure his false and media inspired beliefs and to reverse course toward more pro-social endeavors.

The fact that this teen and millions like him have watched these programs suggests that it cannot be these programs alone that foster negative health behavior. Millions of teens are not turning to deal drugs due to an overly romantic view of the practice.

How do we understand, therefore, who is most vulnerable to emulating what they see in on-screen stories? Clinical practice always involves understanding the uniquely individual ways that culture and biology interact. Because this teen was so influenced by what he was able to watch on TV, it makes sense to consider whether there are other on-screen stories that could just as easily lead to healthier behavior and overall wellbeing. To date, this kind of research has not been systematically conducted. How best to guard against and at the same time to make better use of movies and television programs in the service of clinical care is badly in need of investigation. Whereas the many uses of film for public health initiatives and medical education are increasingly well studied, the utility of film in actual and individual therapeutic endeavors is, unfortunately, still very much lacking.

6

SOLUTIONS TO THE LACK OF ACCESS TO FILM

We have established that film and other forms of on-screen narrative entertainment have positive health uses both inside and outside of a formal healthcare setting. We have also argued that film is perhaps best suited for these endeavors given its ample and relatively inexpensive availability. Still, there are numerous impediments to the enjoyment of cinema and on-screen entertainment. Even though film is arguably one of the least expensive forms of art, it is still costly to many. Home screens cost money. Cable services and movies tickets are increasing in price. Additionally, many disabilities make the appreciation of film more difficult. Traveling to a movie theater can be challenging to those with mobility issues. Vision or hearing problems render this form of art particularly difficult to enjoy. Individuals with autism spectrum syndromes can sometimes feel that they fail to grasp the significance of a given on-screen story that seems obvious to others. Conditions such a stroke, depression, or psychosis can make it hard to understand film. In this chapter, we will examine these impediments and possible work-arounds to allow as many as possible to enjoy film and other forms of on-screen entertainment.

ECONOMIC AND GEOGRAPHICAL LIMITATIONS

The price of movies and cable have steadily risen. Although these data are determined by a variety of factors, including the location that movies or television is available, competing forms of similar or different kinds of entertainment, and pre-existing and sometimes changing social values, most scholars agree that on-screen entertainment is growing less economically feasible for a small subset of the general population. However, there are ample opportunities to work around these limitations. As discussed earlier, community film festivals are increasingly recognized as dependable community-binding forces. Many of these subsidize films that would otherwise not be economically or geographically possible to view. A small community can gain access to obscure films for the purposes of a film festivals, and even larger communities will hold film gatherings to screen movies that are less available in mainstream settings. A study published in the academic journal *Event Management* found that the costs of any film festival must be balanced against the need to make the content of the festival widely available to ensure the success of the gathering (Grunwell, 2007). Additionally, many nations have discounts for both streaming networks and movie tickets for the elderly and for those with disabilities. Finally, free movie screenings, community watch parties for popular television shows and outdoor movies have all been used to help make film more available. Community engagement with popular television has been conceptualized as having a positive effect in community cohesion by making differences such as economic disparities less apparent (Lull, 1980). In addition, the relative ease of access to social media for connection with fans has further facilitated this trend (Guo, 2018).

DISABILITIES AS IMPEDIMENTS
TO THE APPRECIATION OF FILM

Hearing and visual disabilities are two of the largest impediments to the appreciation of home and theater on-screen stories. Studies have found that closed captioning ranks significantly higher than improved hearing aids among older adult who enjoy film and video (Gordon-Salant & Callahan, 2009). For these reasons, closed captioning has become relatively common in streaming networks but ample work-arounds for enjoying movies in the theater are still forthcoming. Some have worried as well that the cost of closed captioning will soon make this service less possible, adding to the already burdensome cost of receiving streaming or broadcast content in the home (Ellcessor, 2012).

For visual impairments, the problems have been harder to tackle. Those who have limited but still present vision can sit near the front of a theater, elect to purchase a high definition screen for the home, or have others explain to them what is taking place on the screen. All of these have their limitations, including decreased comfort, increased costs, and disruptions of others at the theater and at home. Increasingly theaters are providing personalized headsets that describe what is happening on screen, but this practice seems limited to wealthier communities or to art house theaters. For those individuals with visual impairments to truly enjoy cinema, these processes need to become more wide spread. Evidence exists that even graphically complicated images in film can be conveyed through these devices (Walczak, 2017). There is also evidence that many of these devices paradoxically have their instructions written rather than read aloud. One study found that making the simple switch to audio instructions for audio aids would substantially improve the appreciation of movies by those with visual challenges (Romero-Fresco & Fryer, 2013).

Disabilities that affect motility still impair the enjoyment of film both within and outside the home. If a house or apartment is properly outfitted for mechanical assists such as wheelchairs and lifts, then the main impediments occur in theaters. However, the passage of the American with Disabilities Act, and similar laws outside of the United States, have mandated that reasonable accommodations be present outside all facilities where movies are shown. Added services such as public transit that are disability accessible also obviously enhance the ability of those with mobility issues to enjoy films in the theaters (Hastings Comm. & Ent. L.J. 897, 1997–1998).

Finally, we discussed the benefits of film in helping those who suffer psychological challenges to be better understood and to better understand themselves. However, it is also the case that these challenges might make on-screen entertainment harder to appreciate. In these instances, viewers should be encouraged to ask questions about the stories they've watched, and facilitators can even summarize the story before the program or movie begins. These techniques have been effective for conditions such as autism spectrum disorders and for psychotic disorders such as schizophrenia (Emerich, Creaghead, Grether, Murray, & Grasha, 2003; Tsoi et al., 2008).

In some instances, receiving treatment for a given psychological condition is the most effective means by which a film can be understood and appreciated. For example, a significantly depressed person might not be able appreciate all of the nuances and especially the positive affect that a given film has to offer until the depressed mood has abated. On the other hand, there is some evidence that people with depression might actually be more drawn to the consumption of all forms of art. Numerous studies have found that depressed individuals and even individuals who have been in the past significantly depressed are measurably more open to new experiences and especially to new esthetic engagements. The theory in support of these findings is that depressed individuals have a greater chasm between the fantasized self and the true self. To the extent that the fantasized self can be found in art, people with depression might be more drawn to movies, books, painting, and music (Wolfestein & Trull, 1997). However, it is important to note that these findings do not necessarily show that movies and other forms of esthetic consumption are *beneficial* among those who are depressed. Some investigators have found that individuals with depressed affect are indeed more drawn to stories with depressing themes, but there is no sign that absorbing this content helps the person to feel better. This is in potential contrast to the studies cited earlier showing that people who are feeling sad and/or depressed are more likely to and in fact feel better from watching movies with themes of tragedy and sadness. More studies are needed to better delineate to what extent film is beneficial, neutral, or even harmful to those with depression and similar illnesses. For example, there is a school of thought that depression is an evolutionary adaptation to prevent one from wasting energy on largely unobtainable goals (Nesse, 2000). If cinema, through its escapist qualities, takes the place for viewers of what they might in real life try to fruitlessly achieve, then film could be conceptualized as protective against the evolutionary causes of depression itself. On the other hand, viewing others who are able to achieve what the viewer feels are personally hard to reach goals could be alienating and isolating to those whose depression stems from a perception that they have failed at their own, more personal endeavors. It may be that each individual with depression watching a given film will respond differently and in ways that are not easily predicted. In order to draw more consistent conclusions, more studies are needed to establish predictable trends.

7

THE POTENTIAL FOR CINEMA TO UNEXPECTEDLY REDUCE THE STIGMA OF ILLNESS

So far, we have discussed the potential for film to improve sympathy and empathy for illness. We have made the case as well that film holds the potential to increase understanding of the condition of being ill, even for those who have never experienced the illnesses depicted in film. These unique qualities of on-screen narrative entertainment have allowed healthcare professionals to use film in therapeutic, educational, and public health initiatives. We have also argued that these same qualities make film an ideal tool for individuals outside of treatment settings to maintain health and to promote their own well-being. However, there is a very large body of scholarly work noting the ways the films have alienated those with illnesses, creating a self-other divide that is at best neutral and is often seen as harmful. This topic has been central to entire textbooks devoted to the perpetuation of stigma through film, and it is again beyond the scope of this book to summarize this extensive research. Still, it would be untrue to argue that film has not created false impressions of illness, and this is perhaps especially the case with psychosis (Goodwin, 2014).

Classic films like *Psycho*, *Night of the Hunter* and even the slasher films of the 1980s often portray those with psychotic illnesses as dangerously violent. This is in stark contrast to the overwhelming evidence showing that individuals with psychosis are substantially more likely to be victims of violence than perpetrators of harmful acts, and that violence committed by those suffering from psychosis is the same or even less than similar acts in the general population.

Nevertheless, current trends in cinema, and especially within the horror genre, suggesting that depictions of psychosis, leads to dangerous behavior, can actually and somewhat paradoxically reduce stigma. This is due to what scholars of film have referred to as the post-modern movement in horror film and other forms of on-screen horror stories. This final chapter will discuss these new ways of looking at movies, and especially at horror movies, as instruments useful in the reduction of stigma in health care. In order to do this, we must begin by defining what is meant when scholars speak of the "post-modern horror" movement.

Generally speaking, post-modern states of mind posit that there are some phenomena for which no satisfying scientific explanation can be offered. There can be hypotheses and these hypotheses can be tested to some extent, but post-modern thinking by definition states that there is no way of knowing for certain. This is in contrast to more modernist views, wherein explanations for hard to understand occurrences or observations are always possible if not yet realized. With regard to movies, therefore, *Psycho* is decidedly modernist. At the end of the film, the exposition by the psychiatrist explains beyond any doubt the reason for Norman Bates' murderous rage. On the other hand, most film historians point to the late 1960s as the birth of the post-modern horror film. George A. Romero's *Night of the Living Dead* offers no real explanation for the rise of the dead or their desire to eat the living. Mr Romero and others continued this trend as more modern horror stories were told. Bad things simply happen. The French film *Them* or the American film *The Strangers* give no plausible explanation for the frightening home invasions. The perpetrators are neither supernatural nor are they ill in any discernible way. When a soon-to-be victim asks one of the masked attackers in *The Strangers* "why are you doing this to us," the attacker nonchalantly responds "because you were home." For the purposes of horror, it is the lack of explanation that makes the horror more palpable and also seems to attract fans in ways that older forms of horror did not (Pinedo, 1996).

One might be tempted to make the case, therefore, that this post-modern movement in horror movies worsens stigma. After all, if there are no reasons for the invaders in *The Stranger*, then how could we possibly ever understand the internal world of the invaders and take steps toward preventing future recurrences of these kinds of attacks. There is a nihilistic surrender that seems to attract movie-goers but one would be hard pressed to say this nihilism fosters a decrease in stigma (Tudor, 1997).

However, stigma results from an inability or a failure to imagine the condition of the other. To some extent, movies like *The Strangers* show how easy it is for us to fail to place ourselves in another, very different person's shoes. It might seem paradoxical, but asking viewers what the motivations could be in movies where key characters behave inexplicably can actually accentuate the fact that not all behaviors are interpretable in classically psychological ways. When we discussed the film *Helen*, we noted that the film's willingness to resist a psychological interpretation for Helen's depression was noted as a potential tool through which viewers can accept the fact that depression is a sickness that happens de novo and not as a function of past life events. This is a kind of post-modern explanation that therefore serves to reduce stigma rather than accentuate it. *Helen* cannot simply shake off her depression any more than she could shake off a heart attack.

There are even more subtle ways that these post-modern storytelling techniques can be used to decrease stigma. Increasingly, many of the most compelling on-screen horror stories present a potent and even sympathetic sense of ambiguity. Characters who hear the voices of demons might not hear these voices at all; they might simply be suffering from auditory hallucinations. Films such as *They Look Like People* and *The Babadook*, both critically acclaimed movies, benefit precisely because the viewer is never made aware of whether or not the seemingly demonic or psychotic experiences of the protagonists are without question one or the other.

In *They Look Like People*, the protagonist is certain the Earth is being invaded by demonic forces that he can sense but that otherwise look like his fellow human beings. The protagonist is finally "cured" of his fears when his best friend trusts him, even though neither knows for certain whether the concerns of the protagonist are legitimate. Furthermore, the viewer is in much the same predicament. Throughout the film, in every instance where the demons are sensed, the viewer has no reason to doubt the perceptions of the protagonist that demons are in fact present or to doubt the contrary explanation of a medically driven psychosis.

Similarly, in *The Babadook*, the grief of a widowed mother could be the impetus to an intimate and terrifying series of psychotically imagined encounters with a frightening monster, or the monster might in fact truly be present and real. There are literally no scenes in the movie where both explanations are not possible, and the viewer is never told which to believe. Additional movies with these same dilemmas include *Martin*, as well as found footage films like *The Blair Witch Project*. In fact, some have argued that the relatively modern phenomenon of ample video recording devices available to everyday users has made this kind of story telling more plausible (Och, 2015). These so-called found footage films ask a fundamental question: Do we believe what we see on the screen in the theater or what we see on the screen that appears on the screen in the theater? This query can be seen as a metaphor for some of the most basic issues that those with psychotic symptoms face. That is, from a culturally western diagnostic perspective, one does not actually believe that the voices heard by someone who has been diagnosed with a condition characterized by auditory hallucinations actually exist. We might believe that the person with the condition hears these voices, but this is not the same thing as believing the experience of the person himself who hears the voices. Here we need to keep in mind that the beginning of self-other diatheses for stigma derives from our unwillingness to imagine what the person who is stigmatized experiences. In films where it is never clear whether the voices are "real" or present only as hallucinations, viewers might find that they are better able to understand the position of the person who hears the voices in the first place. This understanding can lead to more authentic empathic connection and thus a greater sense of understanding and decreased overall stigma.

These conclusions have led some, including myself, to use some modern horror films as a means of creating empathy for conditions that seem extremely difficult to otherwise understand (Theriot, 2013; https://www.psychologytoday.com/us/blog/grand-rounds/201710/six-horror-films-will-intrigue-psychiatrists). In this way, the ambiguity that the viewer experiences can help to reduce the stigma associated with these illnesses through the development of greater empathy for the shared experiences of the characters on the screen and those who are viewing the story (Byrne, 2009; Rosenstock, 2003). However, this approach can of course backfire. Some might view these interpretations as suggestions that nothing can be done to improve psychosis. Others might choose to interpret the seemingly psychotic symptoms as "proof" of the supernatural. The fact remains, after all, that no one can prove that someone who hears a voice isn't actually hearing something real that no one else is able to hear. This interpretation might therefore serve to negate belief in psychosis in favor of more supernatural explanations, and we have a long and rather sordid history of interpreting psychosis as supernatural and then abusing those whom we have decided that the supernatural afflict. To avoid these kinds of conclusions, clinician-educators should note that most illnesses have at some time been thought to have supernatural or at least superstitious explanations. The lack of a current and coherent explanation does not mean that such an explanation will forever be missing, and it certainly does not provide moral cover for the increased stigma that the lack of a satisfying explanation might otherwise prevent. Furthermore, from a practical point of view, the lack of a clear etiologic understanding does not preclude effective treatments. Psychotic disorders have many remedies that are often extremely successful. In other words, the nihilism of the movies does not necessarily translate to nihilism at the bedside or in the clinician's office. These are important points to stress when one attempts to use these kinds of films as mechanisms to combat stigma.

8

FUTURE DIRECTIONS AND CONCLUSIONS

This book makes the case that film and other forms of on-screen entertainment are among the most ubiquitous forms of art, and that these forms of art also have clear effects on our health. These effects can be positive or negative. Indeed, sometimes the same film has been shown for some to improve health and for others to threaten well-being. This is of course consistent with art in general. It is the rare work of art that is universally celebrated or universally derided. Films and television programs that manage to confer positive or negative health effects do so as a result of an extremely complex interplay of individual tastes, the context in which the on-screen entertainment is consumed, and the methods used to take advantage of what the film has to offer.

Furthermore, film has the capacity to generate greater public health through community cohesion, more effective public educational efforts, and efficient use in the classrooms of those who are studying to practice some form of healthcare delivery. It is not simply the case that any film with a health-related theme is useful. The willingness to utilize film takes a great deal of thought, a willingness to invest substantial creative energy and the patience to engage in the empiricism of trial and error. Perhaps because of the growth of accessibility for virtually all forms of on-screen narrative content, serious academic efforts to study the health effects of film and television programs are relatively recent and still fall far short of being able to generate a cohesive set of guidelines.

These efforts are even more complicated by the rate at which the means of on-screen entertainment is changing. Video games are increasing elaborate and increasingly laden with complex moral and even medical quandaries. Virtual reality has shown promise in the management of chronic pain, in helping those with dementia and even in psychotherapy. The new movement toward the use of psychedelic substances such as MDMA and Ketamine could lead to an entirely new kind of therapy in which researchers will need to discover which films confer even greater therapeutic utility in the presence of powerful psychoactive medications. There will be developments without question in the study of the relationship of film to health that might seem common place in a few decades but that at this point have not even been considered. This is what makes the field of health humanities in general so fascinating, and the possibilities inherent in learning specifically about film and health endlessly intriguing.

However, we must also remember that films themselves are only sometimes made with the viewer's health in mind. Most forms of on-screen storytelling are the product of the explicit desire among the producers to entertain and perhaps to generate revenue from the viewer as well as from sponsors. This means that when we examine the health effects of film, we ought to carefully scrutinize these films for all of the possible motivators that went into the creation of these works of art in the first place. There is, after all, no reason that the agenda of filmmakers and the agenda of those interested in using film to discuss health ought to be the same. However, all forms of art are frequently used for agendas quite different from the intentions of the artists themselves. Because sickness, health, and well-being are integral parts of the human condition, it is likely that there will continue to be a huge swath of on-screen stories from which to draw health-related conclusions. The examples mentioned in this book have only begun to scratch that surface.

Finally, and for goodness sakes, none of this hand-wringing means that we can't enjoy a film for reasons other than its potential effects on our health. The very nature of any humanistic endeavor is its inherent capacity to be absorbed in multiple settings, for multiple reasons, and with a magnificent multitude of results. This is the strength especially for something as ubiquitous as film. But for the purposes of this book, try something new with the next film you watch. Ask yourself, *how does this film affect my health*. You might be surprised at the complexities of your answer.

URL LINKS

http://www.mentalhealthfilmfest.nyc
https://www.nami.org/Blogs/NAMI-Blog/December-2017/
The-Best-Movies-About-Mental-Health
https://smhff.com
https://annenberg.usc.edu/research/aii

REFERENCES

CHAPTER 1

Caputo, N., & Rouner, D. (2011). Narrative processing of entertainment media and mental illness stigma. *Health Communication, 26*(7), 595–604.

Cartwright, L. (2016). Learning from *Philadelphia*: Topographies of HIV/AIDS media assemblages. *Journal of Homosexuality, 63*(3), 369–386.

Fancourt, D., Perkins, R., Ascenso, S., Carvalho, L. A., Steptoe, A., & Williamon, A. (2016). Effects of group drumming interventions on anxiety, depression, social resilience and inflammatory immune response among mental health service users. *PLoS One, 11*(3), e0151136. doi:10.1371/journal.pone.0151136

Schlozman, S. C., Groves, J. E., & Weisman, A. D. (2004). Coping with illness and psychotherapy of the medically ill. In T. A. Stern, G. L. Fricchione, N. H. Cassen, M. S. Jellinek, & J. R. Rosenbaum (Eds.), *Handbook of general hospital psychiatry* (pp. 61–68). Philadelphia, PA: Mosby.

Speer, N., Reynolds, J., Swallow, K., & Zacks, J. (2009, August). Reading stories activates neural representations of visual and motor experiences. *Psychological Science, 20*(8), 989–999.

Tutt, R. (1991). Truth, beauty and travesty: Woody Allen's well wrought urn. *Literature Film Quarterly, 19*(2), 104.

URL Links

https://www.chicagotribune.com/news/ct-xpm-1986-05-11-8602030023-story.html. Accessed on February 9, 2020.

https://www.youtube.com/watch?v=fc0uxTiUDrE. Accessed on February 9, 2020.

CHAPTER 2

Bohnlein, J., Altegoer, L., Kristin, M., Roemann, K., Redlich, R., Dannlowski, U., Leehr, E. J. (2020). Factors influencing the success of exposure therapy for specific phobia: A systematic review. *Neuroscience & Biobehavioral Reviews, 108,* 796–820.

Forssell, R. (2016). Exploring cyberbullying and face-to-face bullying in working life: Prevalence, targets and expressions. *Computers in Human Behavior, 58,* 454–460.

Jones, A. H. (2000). Medicine and the movies: Lorenzo's oil at century's end. *Annals of Internal Medicine, 133*(7), 567–571.

Kite, D., Gullifer, J., & Tyson, G. (2013). Views on the diagnostic labels of autism and Asperger's disorder and the proposed changes in the DSM. *Journal of Autism & Developmental Disorders, 43*(7), 1692–1700.

Nansel, T. R., Overpeck, M., Pilla, R. S., Ruan, W. J., Simons-Morton, B., & Scheidt, P. (2001). Bullying behaviors among US youth. *Journal of the American Medical Association, 285*(16), 2094.

Noam, G. G. (1999). The psychology of belonging: Reformulating adolescent development. In A. H. Esman, L. T. Flaherty, & H. A. Horowitz (Eds.), *Annals of the American society for adolescent psychiatry. Adolescent psychiatry: Development and clinical studies* (Vol. 24, pp. 49–68). Hillsdale, NJ: Analytic Press.

Obermann, M.-L. (2011). Moral disengagement among bystanders to school bullying. *Journal of School Violence, 10*(3), 239–257.

Schmitt, W. J., & Müri, R. M. (2009). Neurobiologie der Spinnenphobie. *Schweizer Archiv für Neurologie, 160*(8), 352–355.

Stern, S. C., & Barnes, J. L. (2019). Brief report: Does watching *The Good Doctor* affect knowledge of and attitudes toward autism? *Journal of Autism and Developmental Disorders, 49,* 2581–2588.

Yahn, M. (2012). The social context of bullying. *Encounter, 25*(4), 20–28.

URL Links

https://ew.com/movies/2018/03/07/reese-witherspoon-wrinkle-in-time. Accessed on February 11, 2020.

https://www.hollywoodreporter.com/features/making-eighth-grade-how-bo-burnham-brought-his-anxiety-screen-1162239. Accessed on February 11, 2020.

https://www.theguardian.com/commentisfree/2018/dec/17/rain-man-myth-autistic-people-dustin-hoffman-savant. Accessed on February 10, 2020.

https://www.youtube.com/watch?v=hJAGxAeV7YU&t=188s. Accessed on February 8, 2020.

https://www.cdc.gov/mmwr/volumes/67/ss/ss6706a1.htm#suggestedcitation. Accessed on February 10, 2020.

Stopbullying.gov. Accessed on February 10, 2020.

CHAPTER 3

Bell, T. R. (2018). Documentary film as collaborative ethnography: Using a thirdspace lens to explore community and race. *Critical Arts: A South-North Journal of Cultural & Media Studies*, 32(5/6), 17–34.

Benet, L., Grout, P., & Dagostino, M. (2009 , September 4). Small towns, big hearts. *People*, 72(11), 84–86.

Drexler, P. (2001). The German courtroom film during the Nazi period: Ideology, aesthetics, historical context. *Journal of Law & Society*, 28(1), 64–78.

Fancourt, D., Williamon, A., Carvalho, L. A., Steptoe, A., Dow, R., & Lewis, I. (2016). Singing modulates mood, stress, cortisol, cytokine and neuropeptide activity in cancer patients and carers. *Ecancermedicalscience*, 10(630–650), 1–13.

Henderson, H., Child, S., Moore, S., Moore, J. B., & Kaczynski, A. T. (2016). The influence of neighborhood aesthetics, safety, and social cohesion on perceived stress in disadvantaged communities. *American Journal of Community Psychology*, 58(1/2), 80–88.

Johns, L., Aiello, A., Cheng, C., Galea, S., Koenen, K., & Uddin, M. (2012). Neighborhood social cohesion and posttraumatic stress disorder in a community-based sample: Findings from the Detroit Neighborhood Health Study. *Social Psychiatry & Psychiatric Epidemiology, 47*(12), 1899–1906.

Khamsi, R. (2005). Laughter boosts blood-vessel health. *Nature* Retrieved from https://www.nature.com/articles/news050307-4#citeas..

Morris, R. V. (2018). Student research: Documentaries made in the community. *Social Studies, 109*(1), 34–44.

Padva, G., & Martyrs, G. (2011). Jewish saints and infatuated Yeshiva boys in the New Israeli Religious queer cinema. *Journal of Modern Jewish Studies, 10*(3), 421–438.

Pearce, E., Launay, J., Machin, A., & Dunbar, R. I. M. (2016). Is group singing special? Health, well-being and social bonds in community-based adult education classes. *Journal of Community & Applied Social Psychology, 26*(6), 518–533.

Scarnato, J. M. (2018). Media production as therapy: A systematic review. *Journal of Technology in Human Services, 36*(4), 241–273.

Weaver, A. J., & Frampton, J. R. (2019). Crossing the color line: An examination of mediators and a social media intervention for racial bias in selective exposure to movies. *Communication Monographs, 86*(4), 399–415.

Webster, A. (2012). The week ahead. *New York Times*, July. Retrieved from https://archive.nytimes.com/query.nytimes.com/gst/fullpage-9A0CEE DC113BF932A35754C0A9649D8B63.html

Yasar, Z. (2019). "Emek is ours, Istanbul is ours": Reimagining a movie theater through urban activism. *Velvet Light Trap: A Critical Journal of Film & Television, 83*, 46–59.

URL Links

https://www.screendaily.com/comment/whats-the-purpose-of-film-festivals-in-the-21st-century/5108598.article. Accessed on February 11, 2020.

https://scienceonscreen.org. Accessed on February 11, 2020.

CHAPTER 4

Bozzuto, J. C. (1975). Cinematic neurosis following "The Exorcist": Report of four cases. *Journal of Nervous and Mental Disease, 161,* 43–48.

Carmichael, V., & Whitley, R. (2018). Suicide portrayal in the Canadian media: Examining newspaper coverage of the popular Netflix series '13 Reasons Why'. *BMC Public Health, 18*(1), 1086.

Huesmann, L. R. (2007). The impact of electronic media violence: Scientific theory and research. *Journal of Adolescent Health, 41*(6 Suppl 1), S6–S13.

Oliver, M. B. (1993, March). Exploring the paradox of the enjoyment of sad films. *Human Communication Research, 19*(3), 315–324.

Schramm, H., & Wirth, W. (2010). Exploring the paradox of sad-film enjoyment: The role of multiple appraisals and meta-appraisals. *Poetics, 38*(3), 319–335.

Strizhakova, Y., & Krcmar, M. (2007). Mood management and video rental choices. *Media Psychology, 10*(1), 91–112.

Till, B., Tran, U. S., Voracek, M., Sonneck, G., & Niederkrotenthaler, T. (2014). Associations between film preferences and risk factors for suicide: An online survey. *PLoS One, 9*(7), e102293.

Tucker, H., Lewis, R. B., Martin, G. L., & Over, C. H. R. (1957). Television therapy: Effectiveness of closed-circuit television as a medium for therapy in treatment of the mentally ill. *AMA Archives of Neurology and Psychiatry, 77*(1), 57–69.

Webb, S. (2010). A corpus driven study of the potential for vocabulary learning through watching movies. *International Journal of Corpus Linguistics, 15*(4), 497–519.

URL Links

https://www.webmd.com/mental-health/features/movie-therapy-using-movies-for-mental-health#1. Accessed on February 11, 2020.

https://www.youtube.com/watch?v=WoYrpA3v-38. Accessed on February 11, 2020.

https://www.youtube.com/watch?v=9-zf2UBp7fY. Accessed on February 11, 2020.

CHAPTER 5

Battles, K., & Hilton-Morrow, W. (2002). Gay characters in conventional spaces: Will and Grace and the situation comedy genre. *Critical Studies in Media Communication, 19*(1), 87–105.

Baumann, S. E., Merante, M., Folb, B. L., & Burke, J. G. (2020). Is film as a research tool the future of public health? A review of study designs, opportunities, and challenges. *Qualitative Health Research, 30*(2), 250–2570.

Bhagar, H. A. (2005). Should cinema be used for medical student education in psychiatry? *Medical Education, 39*(9), 972–973.

Calvert, S. L., & Tart, M. (1993). Song versus verbal forms for very-long-term, long-term, and short-term verbatim recall. *Journal of Applied Developmental Psychology, 14*(2), 245–260.

Duffy, A., Dawson, D. L., & das Nair, R. (2016, May). Pornography addiction in adults: A systematic review of definitions and reported impact. *The Journal of Sexual Medicine, 13*(5), 760–777.

Elman, J. P. (2010). After school special education: Rehabilitative television, teen citizenship, and compulsory able-bodiedness. *Television & New Media, 11*(4), 260–292.

Flores, G. (2004). Doctors in the movies. *Archives of Disease in Childhood, 89*, 1084–1088.

Hall, R. C., & Friedman, S. H. (2015). Psychopathology in a Galaxy far, far away: The use of star wars' dark side in teaching. *Academic Psychiatry, 39*(6), 726–732.

Hickey, C. (2018). Freud and frozen: Using film to teach psychodynamic psychotherapy. *Journal of Spirituality in Mental Health, 20*(1), 1–13. doi:10.1080/19349637.2017.1314209

Huesmann, L. R. (2007). The impact of electronic media violence: Scientific theory and research. *Journal of Adolescent Health*, *41*(6 Suppl 1), S6–S13.

Jayakaran, T. G., Rekha, C. V., Annamalai, S., Baghkomeh, P. N., & Sharmin, D. D. (2017). Preferences and choices of a child concerning the environment in a pediatric dental operatory. *Dental Research Journal (Isfahan)*, *14*(3), 183–187.

Keeler, A. R. (2016). Premature adulthood: Alcoholic moms and teenage adults in the ABC *Afterschool Specials*. *Quarterly Review of Film and Video*, *33*(6), 483–500.

Kerimoglu, B., Neuman, A., Paul, J., Stefanov, D. G., & Twersky, R. (2003). Anesthesia induction using video glasses as a distraction tool for the management of preoperative anxiety in children. *Anesthesia and Analgesia*, *117*(6), 1373–1379.

Kinner, E. A., & Belmont, M. J. (1993). Motivation in the classroom: Reciprocal effects of teacher behavior and student engagement across the school year. *Journal of Educational Psychology*, *85*(4), 571–581.

Koushiou, M., Nicolaou, K., & Karekla, M. (2018). Inducing negative affect using film clips with general and eating disorder-related content. *Eating and Weight Disorders*, *23*(6), 775–784.

Larsen, J. T., McGraw, A. P., & Cacioppo, J. T. (2001). Can people feel happy and sad at the same time? *Journal of Personality and Social Psychology*, *81*(4), 684–696.

Levin, H. W., & Schlozman, S. (2006). Napoleon dynamite: Asperger's disorder or Geek NOS? *Academic Psychiatry*, *30*, 430–435.

Linn, S. (2003). Children and commercial culture: Expanding the advocacy roles of professionals in education, health, and human service. *Journal of Negro Education*, *72*(4), 478–486.

Marini, M. G. (2016). The place of illness-centred movies in medical humanities. In *Narrative medicine* : Bridging the Gap between Evidence-Based Care and Medical Humanities (pp. 71-80). Switzerland: Springer. https://link.springer.com/content/pdf/bfm%3A978-3-319-22090-1%2F1.pdf.

Millett, C., Polansky, J. R., & Glantz, S. A. (2011). Government inaction on ratings and government subsidies to the US film industry help promote youth smoking. *PLoS Medicine*, 8(8), e1001077.

Nam, S. S., Cha, J. H., & Sung, K. (2019). Connected in cinema: Educational effects of filmmaking classes on medical students. *Korean Journal of Medical Education*, 31(4), 319–330.

Ovetz, R. (2011). Rocking the Schoolhouse: Re-reading "Schoolhouse Rock!" in the college classroom. *Radical Teacher*, 90, 73–74.

Perciaccante, A., Charlier, P., Coralli, A., Deo, S., Appenzeller, O., & Bianucci, R. (2019). Exploring disease representation in movies. *Journal of General Internal Medicine*, 34(11), 2351–2354.

Pike, K. (2011). Lessons in liberation: Schooling girls in feminism and femininity in 1970s ABC Afterschool Specials. *Girlhood Studies*, 4, 95–11.

Schlozman, S. C. (2000). Vampires and those who slay them. *Academic Psychiatry*, 24, 49–54.

Schulenberg, S. E. (2003). Psychotherapy and movies: On using films in clinical practice. *Journal of Contemporary Psychotherapy*, 33, 35–48.

Taylor Williams, S. (2012). "Holy PTSD, Batman!": An analysis of the psychiatric symptoms of Bruce Wayne. *Academic Psychiatry*, 36, 252–255.

Till, B., Tran, U. S., Voracek, M., Sonneck, G., & Niederkrotenthaler, T. (2014). Associations between film preferences and risk factors for suicide: An online survey. *PLoS One*, 9(7), e102293.

Unknown Author. (2016). Adult film ratings to stop kids lighting up. *Bulletin of the World Health Organization*, 94(2), 82–83. doi:10.2471/BLT.16.020216

van Agt, H. M., Korfage, I. J., & Essink-Bot, M. L. (2014). Interventions to enhance informed choices among invitees of screening programmes: A systematic review. *Europena Journal of Public Health*, 24(5), 789–801.

Wilson, N., Heath, D., Heath, T., Gallagher, P., & Huthwaite, M. (2014). Madness at the movies: Prioritised movies for self-directed learning by medical students. *Australasian Psychiatry*, 22(5), 450–453.

URL Links

https://scienceonscreen.org. Accessed on February 11, 2020.

https://www.youtube.com/watch?v=ZzrMrglib6c. Accessed on February 11, 2020.

CHAPTER 6

Ellcessor, E. (2012). Captions on, off, on TV, online: Accessibility and search engine optimization in online closed captioning. *Television & New Media, 13*(4), 329–352.

Emerich, D. M., Creaghead, N. A., Grether, S. M., Murray, D., & Grasha, C. (2003). The comprehension of humorous materials by adolescents with high-functioning autism and Asperger's syndrome. *Journal of Autism & Developmental Disorders, 33*(3), 25.

Gordon-Salant, S., & Callahan, J. S. (2009, August). The benefits of hearing aids and closed captioning for television viewing by older adults with hearing loss. *Ear and Hearing, 30*(4), 458–465.

Grunwell, S. (2007). "Steve" Ha, Inhyuck. *Event Management, 11*(4), 201–210.

Guo, M. (2018). How television viewers use social media to engage with programming: The social engagement scale development and validation. *Journal of Broadcasting & Electronic Media, 62*(2), 195–214.

Hastings Comm. & Ent. L.J. 897. (1997–1998). Down in front: Entertainment facilities and disabled access under the Americans with Disabilities Act.

Lull, J. (1980, March). The social uses of television. *Human Communication Research, 6*(3), 197–209.

Nesse, R. M. (2000). Is depression an adaptation? *Archives of General Psychiatry, 57*(1), 14–20.

Romero-Fresco, P., & Fryer, L. (2013). Could audio-described films benefit from audio introductions? An audience response study. *Journal of Visual Impairment & Blindness, 107*(4), 287–295.

Tsoi, D. T.-Y., Lee, K.-H., Gee, K. A., Holden, K. L., Parks, R. W., & Woodruff, P. W. R. (2008). Humour experience in schizophrenia: Relationship with executive dysfunction and psychosocial impairment. *Psychological Medicine*, *38*(6), 801–810.

Walczak, A. (2017). Creative description: Audio describing artistic films for individuals with visual impairments. *Journal of Visual Impairment & Blindness*, *111*(4), 387–391.

Wolfestein, M., & Trull, T. J. (1997). Depression and openness to experience. *Journal of Personality Assessment*, *69*(3), 614.

CHAPTER 7

Byrne, P. (2009). Why psychiatrists should watch films (or What has cinema ever done for psychiatry?)? *Advances in Psychiatric Treatment*, *15*(4), 286–296.

Goodwin, J. (2014). The horror of stigma: Psychosis and mental health care environments in twenty-first-century horror film (Part II). *Perspectives in Psychiatric Care*, *50*(4), 224–234.

Och, D. (2015). Beyond surveillance: Questions of the real in the neopostmodern horror film. In W. Clayton (Eds.), *Style and form in the Hollywood Slasher film* (pp. 195–212). London: Palgrave Macmillan.

Pinedo, I. (1996). Recreation terror: Postmodern elements of the contemporary horror film. *Journal of Film and Video*, *48*(½, Spring–Summer), 17–31.

Rosenstock, J. (2003). Beyond a beautiful mind: Film choices for teaching psychosis. *Academic Psychiatric*, *27*(2), 117–112.

Theriot, M. T. (2013). Using popular media to reduce New College Students' Mental Illness Stigma. *Social Work in Mental Health*, *11*(2), 118–140.

Tudor, A. (1997). Why horrror? The peculiar pleasures of a popular genre. *Cultural Studies*, *11*(3), 443–463.

URL Links

https://www.psychologytoday.com/us/blog/grand-rounds/201710/six-horror-films-will-intrigue-psychiatrists. Accessed on February 8, 2020.

INDEX